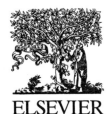

ELSEVIER

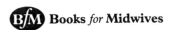 **Books** *for* **Midwives**

  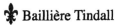

CHURCHILL LIVINGSTONE **Mosby** **THE PRACTISING MIDWIFE** **Baillière Tindall**

MIDWIFERY PUBLISHERS OF CHOICE FOR GENERATIONS

For many years and through several identities we have catered for professional needs in midwifery education and practice. Leading publishers of major textbooks such as *Myles Textbook for Midwives* and *Mayes' Midwifery: a Textbook for Midwives*, our expertise spreads across both books and journals to offer a comprehensive resource for midwives at all stages of their careers.

Find out how we can provide you with the right book at the right time by exploring our website, **www.elsevierhealth.com/midwifery** or requesting a midwifery catalogue from Health Professions Marketing, Elsevier, 32 Jamestown Road, Camden, London, NW1 7BY, UK Tel: 020 7424 4200; Fax: 020 7424 4420.

We are always keen to expand our midwifery list so if you have an idea for a new book please contact Mary Seager, Senior Commissioning Editor at Elsevier, The Boulevard, Langford Lane, Kidlington, Oxford, OX5 1GB, UK (m.seager@elsevier.com).

 Have you joined yet?
Sign up for e-Alert to get the latest news and information.

Register for eAlert at www.elsevierhealth.com/eAlert Information direct to your Inbox

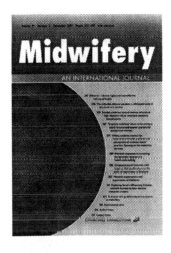

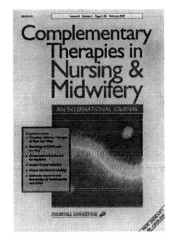

HEALTH PROMOTION IN MIDWIFERY

For Baillière Tindall:

Publishing Manager: Inta Ozols
Project Development Manager: Karen Gilmour
Project Manager: Derek Robertson
Design Direction: George Ajayi

HEALTH PROMOTION IN MIDWIFERY

A Resource for Health Professionals

Jacqueline Dunkley

Senior Lecturer in Midwifery
School of Health, Biological and Environmental Sciences
Middlesex University, London

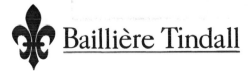

Baillière Tindall

EDINBURGH LONDON NEW YORK OXFORD PHILADELPHIA ST LOUIS SYDNEY TORONTO 2000

BAILLIÈRE TINDALL
An imprint of Elsevier Limited

First published 2000
    Reprinted 2004, 2005

ISBN 0 7020 2424 4

British Library Cataloguing in Publication Data
A catalogue record for this book is available from the British Library

Library of Congress Cataloguing in Publication Data
A catalogue record for this book is available from the Library of Congress

Note
Medical knowledge is constantly changing. As new information becomes available, changes in treatment, procedures, equipment and the use of drugs become necessary. The editors, contributor and the publishers have taken care to ensure that the information given in this text is accurate and up to date. However, readers are strongly advised to confirm that the information, especially with regard to drug usage, complies with the latest legislation and standards of practice.

The Publisher

ELSEVIER your source for books, journals and multimedia in the health sciences
www.elsevierhealth.com

Working together to grow
libraries in developing countries

www.elsevier.com | www.bookaid.org | www.sabre.org

ELSEVIER   BOOK AID International   Sabre Foundation

The
publisher's
policy is to use
**paper manufactured
from sustainable forests**

Printed in China

Contents

Preface

The aim of this book is to highlight the scope of health promotion within midwifery practice and emphasise the unique opportunity midwives have to influence the health and lifestyles of women and their families. The initial chapters present an overview of health and health promotion, and explore this from the midwife's perspective. Inequality in health and health care is an integral part of this section. The subsequent chapters continue the theme of health promotion and its application to midwifery practice. The book should be read sequentially, to enable the reader to utilise an effective and efficient approach to health promotion work. The philosophy of health promotion reflected throughout the following pages is concerned with empowering people to make healthy lifestyle choices, within the context of their cultural and socioeconomic backgrounds.

The government's commitment to increasing health potentials, particularly for those who are disadvantaged, is a commonly reflected theme. However, the scope of health promotion within midwifery practice is not only undervalued but is not supported with the same ambition and rigor as other aspects of clinical work. Pregnancy may be the only time in a woman's life where she has regular contact with a health professional whose focus is on supporting and encouraging health-enhancing behaviours. Midwives are therefore in a unique position to contribute to the future health of society. The benefits of health promotion in midwifery can be gained only if commitment, time and resource allocation are provided. The new political agenda promises this commitment. *Our Healthier Nation, a contract for health* (Secretary of State for Health 1998) emphasises the need for collaboration and partnership between the National Health Service (NHS), local authorities and local communities, with the ultimate aim of reducing inequalities in health by increasing the health of disadvantaged groups.

Reference

Secretary of State for Health 1998 Our healthier nation, a contract for health. A consultation paper. The Stationery Office, London.

Acknowledgements

I would like to dedicate this book to my mother and father who have showered me with support, motivation and love. Their overwhelming commitment and belief in me continues to influence my life both personally and professionally. I express my gratitude to my fiancé who has patiently completed his journey with me and provided an abundance of emotional support. Lastly a warm and hearty thank you to my brother, sisters, friends and colleagues, who have continued to inspire and support me during this challenging period of my life.

Rethinking the concept of health

1

Key themes

- Meanings of health: personal and cultural
- Illness
- Healthy pregnancy
- Holistic health
- Inequalities in health and health care; inequalities in health, women and midwifery
- Health of the nation
- Social justice

Overview

Understanding the meaning of health and its broad interpretations enables an effective and efficient approach to health promotion work. The aim of this chapter is to encourage the reader to re-examine individual and professionally determined ideas about health and factors which influence ill health. Inequalities in health and health care continue to exist today. Despite the wider political and economic contribution to reducing inequality this continues to challenge the government and health agencies. Each health profession has a responsibility to ensure equality for the provision of health care. Strategies for reducing inequalities in health will form the basis of the discussion, enabling a clear and focused starting point for health promotion work. By rethinking the concept of health the reader should reflect on factors which have determined health and illness and critically approach the broader meaning of what being 'healthy' means to clients or patients. Seedhouse (1986), suggests that, 'Everyone involved with health in any way should attempt a personal clarification of the meaning of the word' (p. 25).

The reader may also reflect on the current health care system, which supports objective parameters of Western ideologies of health as determinants of health.

Health and illness

The meanings of health have changed considerably over the last two decades; they have progressed from being defined as the absence of disease toward the recognition that health has a much broader meaning. Lay perspectives on health are influenced by culture, ethnicity, social class, religion, gender and economic status. Medical perspectives on health may focus on the congruent functioning of the organs of a body in the absence of disease. Social scientists may view health as people's ability to function within their culturally determined social customs and norms. Lay healers may view health as the individual's ability to have an harmonious balance between the mind, body and spirit. Beliefs about health undoubtedly influence the maintenance of health, health promotion strategies and the actions of health professionals when seeking to prevent ill health. Being cured by the medic may seem the more favourable option to achieving 'optimum' health, as opposed to being given the tools to live a happy and comfortable life in one's own environment as proposed by the social scientist (Downie, Tannahill & Tannahill 1996).

The World Health Organization (WHO) defines health as: 'a state of complete physical, mental and social well being and not merely the absence of disease or infirmity' (WHO 1946). This definition is well known for broadening the understanding of health during that period of time. Acknowledging physical, mental and social well being broadens the focus of the determinants of health and also implies that strategies to improve health cannot rely upon a medical approach to health and health care. To be in a state of complete physical, mental and social well being, however, is unrealistic, as factors which influence health are not static. Also complete states of health are open to subjective impressions and are relative in nature.

Personal constructs of health and illness vary between individuals and cultures. Biological experiences of health and illness are deeply routed in attitudes and beliefs which form the understanding and interpretation of illness and well being. In an attempt to promote health by encouraging people to consider the health benefits of well-spaced pregnancies and reducing the number of pregnancies, the men in Dassa-Zoume, Benin, were asked what they thought about the health of their wives and children. One based his wife's health on the premise that waking up in the morning defines health. Another felt that the food the woman eats and the pleasure she derives from her children influenced health. Others related women's health to antenatal care during pregnancy, stating this as assuring good health (Safe Motherhood 1996).

Blaxter & Patterson (1982) found that sufferers of multiple sclerosis did not accept that they had lost their good health although suffering from some of the debilitating effects of the illness. Sufferers emphasised that their focus was on activity, keeping going and a positive state of mind.

Different cultural ideas about health often influence a woman's willingness to do, for example, breast self-examinations and therefore benefit from appropriate screening. It may be culturally unacceptable to perform examinations of this nature. A fatalistic attitude has also been a contributory factor in reducing the uptake of screening. Ellerman (1998) suggests that many black women who experience socioeconomic disadvantage in the United States believe that breast cancer ends in a mastectomy and death and are therefore less likely to examine themselves and attend for screening. Similarly American Indian women fear that if they talk about a disease they will contract it. Superstition serves to influence health beliefs.

Reflection points

- What does being healthy mean to you?
- How would you define a healthy pregnancy?
- Would your definition of a healthy pregnancy be the same as your definition of a healthy pregnant mother?

You're not ill, you're just pregnant!

Ill health can be described as physical and/or mental states which inhibit individuals from functioning to their 'normal' potential. Ill health may be based on individual perception or professionally determined criteria. Feelings of ill health may not be classed as illness if there are no significant clinical signs. During pregnancy illness traits may be considered 'normal' responses to a 'natural' process. A pregnant woman is considered to be in good health if she is physically and mentally well adjusted to the pregnancy, with no adverse maternal or fetal risk factors. The woman is also expected to 'bloom' during middle to late pregnancy, displaying signs of health and well being. This common stereotype, perpetuated by society, may inhibit women from verbalising their feelings and responses to the physiological adjustment taking place. Signs and symptoms and general feelings of ill health which seek to inform individual knowledge about pregnancy and birth may be suppressed. Distorted body image, including weight gain, breast enlargement and striae gravidarum, may challenge individual ideas about sexuality and cause psychological trauma in some women, whilst others may feel empowered by such changes.

A pregnancy which progresses without medical intervention is viewed as 'normal'. Similarly, disorders of pregnancy are considered to be 'normal' and positively welcomed by some as an indication that the pregnancy is advancing well. For instance, nausea and vomiting, heartburn, constipation, haemorrhoids, varicose veins, backache, swollen feet and ankles, carpal tunnel syndrome and general aches and pains are common disorders of pregnancy and are primarily the result of increased weight gain and hormonal adjustment necessary for the maintenance of the pregnancy. They vary in their occurrence and severity but do not constitute ill health. Disorders which increase in severity, including the development of hyperemesis gravidarum, constitute illness, this condition poses a threat to maternal and fetal health.

The major medical attempt to increase well being during pregnancy had catastrophic consequences. In the early 1960s thalidomide, a sedative and tranquilliser, was prescribed for women during the first trimester of pregnancy for relief of nausea and vomiting. The use of the drug was, however, terminated when evidence suggested that the drug was the cause of congenital malformations.

Advice, empathy and support are strategies commonly used by midwives to help women relieve the effects of the disorders of pregnancy. Medical referral is unlikely, unless the disorder becomes excessive and poses a threat to the health of the mother and fetus. The woman may feel ill both physically and mentally yet her symptoms may still be considered to lie within the realms of normality. In contrast, if the disorders listed were experienced by a non-pregnant woman, the root cause thus removed, the symptoms would be categorised as ill health and warrant further medical investigation. Pregnancy is often termed as 'healthy', 'progressing well' or 'normally'. The woman however, may not be progressing 'normally' as her experiences of the disorders of pregnancy may feel very abnormal and challenge her concept of health and illness. She may not consider herself to be in a state of complete physical, mental and social health, but because she is pregnant her feelings may be somewhat dismissed or summarised into plausible explanations that render her experiences meaningless.

In contrast to the feelings of ill health, women who suffer from pre-eclampsia are renowned for feeling well despite the presence of the disease, which is medically defined as potentially life-threatening. Concepts of health and illness therefore extend far beyond medical explanation. Attempts to define health based on this example may therefore be futile in providing a watertight definition. Reassurance of 'normality' may, however, alleviate anxiety and worry, by enabling the woman to understand that the symptoms are a response to a normal process. Illness is a subjective experience of loss of health. It is described by Naidoo & Wills (1998) as the presentation of symptoms of, for example, aches and pains or loss of function, but if the cause of the problem during pregnancy is considered a normal physiological response the woman is not categorised as being ill; she is just pregnant! This obvious contradiction in terms serves only to reinforce the benefits of the individualised approach to care during pregnancy and the continued need for empathy and understanding when subjective impressions of illness are made, regardless of the cause. The woman is often reacting to her subjective experience of pregnancy, and her feelings and emotions which accompany this event. Graham & Oakley (1986) give similar examples from research projects, which are concerned with medical and maternal perspectives on pregnancy in which women describe health and illness during pregnancy not only from a physiological perspective but also from a social perspective.

I am not attempting to liken pregnancy to illness as midwives have spent many decades trying to relinquish pregnancy from the sick role, after a series of government committees, Cranbrook (Report of the Maternity Services Committee 1959) and then Peel (DHSS 1970). Both made recommendations for childbirth to take place in the hospital, encouraging the medicalisation of childbirth and thus the adoption of the sick role. It is purely my intention to broaden the scope for understanding health and anticipating problems which may occur when health promotion strategies are utilised in later chapters.

It is evident so far that physical, mental and social facets of health are interlinked. Initiatives which aim to promote physical well being, to the exclusion of mental and social facets of health, may therefore prove ineffective.

Health as an holistic concept

Health described as an holistic concept refers to all dimensions of health including its physical, mental, emotional, societal, sexual and spiritual aspects. An awareness and appreciation of the dimensions should not encourage one dimension of health to be viewed independently of the others. They are inextricably linked, therefore a deficit in one dimension affects another or all other dimensions. All aspects of health are interrelated and interdependent (Ewles & Simnett 1999).

Box 1.1 **Case study: Michelle**

Michelle is 22 weeks' pregnant and continues to have nausea and vomiting throughout the morning only. She works for an agency and as such does not get paid sick or holiday pay. She is the sole wage earner in the family and has two children and a partner to support. Unfortunately she has not been able to work as consistently as she would like and cannot get work in the afternoons only, when the nausea and vomiting have subsided. She is extremely worried and anxious about falling behind on bill payments, having enough money to feed the family as well as save money for travel into work if she is able. She knows that if she is not consistent with her working arrangements with the agency, they may not give her work when she is able. She becomes very angry and frustrated toward her partner and they argue frequently. In an attempt to maintain the finances, Michelle compromises her health by feeding the children but not eating herself. Her fluid intake also reduces and she finds it difficult to sleep at night owing to worry. She described herself as feeling depressed and under pressure. She was ultimately admitted to hospital diagnosed with dehydration and a urine infection. Michelle progressed to deliver a 1.8 kg baby at 38 weeks' gestation, whom she described as healthy and well.

Consider the case study in Box 1.1. Societal health refers to health and the way society is structured (Naidoo & Wills 1998). In the scenario above Michelle's health was compromised due to an inability to meet and maintain basic physiological needs. Maslow (1954) suggests that human needs are organised in a hierarchy where physiological needs represent the bottom of the hierarchy and must be satisfied before an individual can seek to address higher needs such as safety, belonging, self-esteem, intellectual and aesthetic needs and finally, at the top of the hierarchy, self-actualisation.

Michelle's mental health began to deteriorate as she was unable to think clearly and coherently; this affected her emotional and social health, which are inextricably linked, her physical health inevitably suffered and she was admitted to hospital with an illness. Emotional distress can lead to physical illness by affecting the immune response (Sutherland & Cooper 1990). Michelle, however, was not in a state of health at the beginning of the scenario. This situation is not uncommon, some mothers compromise their diet to enable their offspring to eat, due to socioeconomic disadvantage (Dobson et al 1994, Dowler & Calvert 1995).

Furthermore Michelle's description of a healthy, well baby is determined by the association made within the context of the present moment. It is well documented that babies who are of low birth weight are at increased risk of cardiovascular disease and related disorders in later life (Barker 1998).

A philosophical approach to the meaning of health

In an attempt to clarify the meaning of health, Seedhouse (1986) explores the concept of health from a philosophical perspective. Seedhouse offers a theory of health which suggests that 'a person's health is equivalent to the state of the set of conditions which fulfil or enable a person to work to fulfil his or her realistic chosen and biological potentials' (p. 72). This view of health infers that those who work to promote health should recognise or facilitate the recognition of the individual's chosen and biological potential and tailor the health promotion approach to function within this context. Integral to this approach would be the provision of basic means by which chosen goals can be achieved. This view of health involves empowering people and enabling the growth of an individual or groups to achieve their health potentials whilst recognising the socioeconomic and political arena which serves to weaken the foundations for some members of society. The theory may, however, present a misconception that the biological and chosen potential of a working class woman on income support can achieve only what is available and accessible within her disadvantaged framework. It is suggested that people can progress beyond class distinctions but chosen biological potentials must be the focus for progression. Seedhouse seeks to clarify negative ideas about the theory by challenging ideas that health for all can be achieved. He suggests that this notion is purely utopian and instead offers a realistic view of health which is based on individual potentials. This theory leaves little room for the creation of false hope and subsequent disappointment.

By critically exploring several theories of health (Box 1.2), Seedhouse recognises a common aim and states that despite conflicts between theories and their different meanings of health they share the common factor of working toward acknowledging the conditions necessary for the achievement of biological and chosen potentials.

I have willed to go forward and have not advanced beyond the borders of my grave

(Saniya Salih, Syrian poet 1985)

Discussion questions

- Consider the theories of health presented in Figure 2.1 (p. 36).
- What are the problems implicit when embracing each theory?

Inequalities in health

The overall health of the population may have improved but the improvement is at present predominantly among the higher social classes. Inequalities in health are still evident today; social and economic disadvantage results in the poorer members of society remaining in poor housing, experiencing unemployment and suffering from stress (Acheson 1998, Office for National Statistics 1998, Whitehead 1988). The majority of diseases and the highest mortality rates are still found in areas of deprivation and disadvantage amongst the least affluent members of society (Research Unit in Health and Behavioural Change 1989, Secretary of State for Health 1999). Focus on the individual to prevent ill health will not only be ineffective in reducing levels of disease and encouraging healthy lifestyles but also disguises the social, economic and environmental issues which predispose vulnerability to disease and illness (Research Unit in Health and Behavioural Change 1989). Although individual counselling encourages one in four of those who participate to make health-related behavioural change, those who are most likely to fail and have least motivation to change are the least well off and the poorer members of society (Gillies &

Box 1.2 **The theories of health**

- The theory that health is an ideal state
- The theory that health is the physical and mental fitness to do socialised daily tasks
- The theory that health is a commodity which can be brought or given
- A group of theories which hold that health is a personal strength or ability, whether physical, metaphysical or intellectual

---

Spray 1997). Health promotion strategies directed toward the broader social, environmental and economical issues may be more effective at helping and supporting all members of the community. The focus of this is quite clearly political.

Government action to reduce inequalities – an overview

Inequalities in health have existed for centuries and are sure to exist throughout the twenty-first century. Discussions to reduce inequalities in health have taken place at levels of political and social theory. An outward display of the unacceptable growing levels of inequality in health was made to the government, which led to the publication of the well-known Black report in 1980 (Black et al 1982). This report clearly showed that the major determinants of health were concerned with social class, economic conditions, geographical location and gender. People in the upper socioeconomic classes were more likely to avoid illness and stay healthy than those of the lower socioeconomic classes. Sir Douglas Black and colleagues suggested government intervention, recommendations and further research into the causes of social inequalities in health. Despite alarming but not surprising findings, the recommendations were not endorsed as the cost involved was estimated at £2 billion per year at 1980's inflation rate. Positive outcomes of the report may be implied by the stimulation of extensive international research into inequalities in health (Dovey et al 1990, Townsend, Davidson & Whitehead 1992).

The pre-election promise in 1997 by the new Labour Government included an independent review into the inequalities in health, which advanced 39 recommendations (Acheson 1998). The report urges the government to implement the recommendations in order to promote social justice. It does not, however, detail the process of implementation or costing. Recommendations include:

- enabling women with families who wish to combine working with parenting to do so, by removing barriers to participation and the provision of affordable accessible childcare
- increasing benefits to reduce the level of poverty
- development of policies which improve the nutritional health of women of childbearing age and their families
- development of policies which increase the accessibility and affordability of foodstuff
- development of policies which will increase the prevalence of breast feeding

Discussion questions

- Consider the recommendations of the Acheson report (1998).
- How will they impact on the users of maternity services?
- What is the role of the midwife in the implementation of the recommendations?

- effective programmes that will enable pregnant mothers to give up smoking
- development of policies that will promote the social and emotional support for expectant parents.

The white paper, Saving lives, our healthier nation (Secretary of State for Health 1999), acknowledges the recommendations of the independent inquiry into the inequalities in health and proposes to reduce inequalities. Its key aims are:

To improve the health of the population as a whole by increasing the length of people's lives and the number of years people spend free from illness.

To improve the health of the worst off in society and to narrow the health gap.

(Secretary of State for Health 1999)

Its intent is to focus government action on social and environmental areas that damage people's lives. Unlike the Health of the nation report, where the focus of attention was on individual responsibility to prevent poor health (DOH 1992), the 1999 white paper acknowledges that the cause of ill health does not rest solely with individuals. Blaming the individual for not taking advice to improve their health is not a focus of this report. The government proposes a contract for better health which sets out responsibilities for improving health, the focus of which is on the 'new public health'. The emphasis, however, is on everyone playing a part including the government, those at national level, communities, families and individuals. The document recognises that improvements in health can only be achieved by a combined top-down (government) and bottom-up (community) approach and commitment. Identified target areas to be achieved by the year 2010 include reductions in heart disease and stroke, accidents, cancer and improved mental health. The proposed targets may, however, be viewed by some as a public relations exercise demonstrating the government's commitment to reducing inequalities in health but with little action. Until the written contract becomes a working reality this commitment from the government may be viewed as a platitude for gaining acceptance and support. Others argue that, by proposing the devolvement of responsibility for health improvements to local authorities, the government is avoiding its responsibility to give national leadership (Horton 1998). Downie, Tannahill & Tannahill (1996) suggest that targets should be viewed as a means of achieving progress toward improving quality of life, not as an end in themselves.

Health of the nation

A useful indicator of the nation's health is the falling infant mortality rate since the early part of the twentieth century. The fall is projected to continue by a further 57% by the year 2021, based on 1996 infant mortality rates. The fall in infant mortality has contributed to the improvement of life expectancy at birth. This has increased by 60% in England and Wales since the turn of the twentieth century and is currently increasing by 2 years every decade. Although these figures are reassuring the increase in life expectancy does not necessarily mean a healthy life. Research carried out by the University of Kent (England), found that healthy life expectancy remained almost constant between 1976 and 1994, at approximately 59 years for males and 62 years for females. Total life expectancy at birth rose during this period from approximately 70 to 75 years for males and from 76 to 80 years for females (see Table 1.1.). This suggests that the extra years of life gained by the elderly may not necessarily mean *healthy* life (Office for National Statistics 1998).

Inequalities in health, women and midwifery

Midwives contribute to the health of the nation and have an important contribution to make to women's health. In the United Kingdom deaths from childbirth are rare. The maternal mortality rate between 1994 and 1996 is reported to be 12.2 per 100 000 maternities (Department of Health (DOH) 1998). A death rate from pregnancy-related illness or births is reported to be as high as 437 per 100 000 maternities in India, with three-quarters noted as preventable (Royal College of Midwives (RCM) 1997). Basic needs including sanitation, immunisation and adequate nutrition as well as poor provision of, and accessibility to, health care are major determinants of mortality. Poor diet and health during pregnancy results in sick babies who may among other complications be growth retarded during uterine life and have an increased mortality and morbidity in the first year of life (Vit et al 1996), and throughout

Table 1.1 Life expectancy[1] and healthy life expectancy at birth: by gender, England & Wales		1901	1971	1976	1981	1985	1991	1994	1996
Males									
	Life expectancy	45.3	69.0	70.0	71.1	71.9	73.4	74.3	74.6
	Healthy life expectancy	–	–	58.3	58.7	58.8	59.9	59.2	–
Females									
	Life expectancy	49.2	75.2	76.1	77.1	77.6	78.9	79.6	79.7
	Healthy life expectancy	–	–	62.0	61.0	61.9	63.0	62.2	–

Reproduced with the permission of 'Social trends 28', Office of National Statistics © Crown copyright 1998.
[1]See Appendix, Part 7: Expectation of life.

childhood (Middle et al 1996). This startling reality of inequality between nations is clearly a political issue. Women's health issues must remain high on the political agenda if the deaths from childbirth are ever to reduce in the developing countries. It is suggested that midwives should continue as far as possible to bring to the attention of politicians the factors which will improve the health of women and subsequently their reproductive success (Thompson 1996). Focusing on data presented closer to home, within the United Kingdom, babies of women in disadvantaged groups are more likely to have suffered from intrauterine growth retardation. Also babies of fathers who are in disadvantaged groups have birth weights of 130 g lower than babies of fathers who are socioeconomically advantaged (Office for National Statistics 1998).

The maternal mortality rate in many countries of central and eastern Europe is up to ten times higher than in many Western countries of the European region. The World Health Organization suggests that an emerging response and long term investment are needed if the trends are to be reversed. The conference on the health of women in central Europe (WHO 1997) identified and agreed priority action areas which include:

- to upgrade maternal and child health services
- to promote breast feeding
- to update the knowledge and skills of midwives
- to protect against inappropriate medical technology
- to promote programmes emphasising healthy lifestyles and programmes to reduce violence against women. In order to strengthen the commitment to women's health in policy reform it was suggested that more women should be appointed to leadership positions and be instrumental in ensuring the involvement of women's groups in policy development.

Inequalities in the provision of midwifery health care

Selective visiting

Both postnatal and antenatal selective visiting are based on client need and clinical judgement. The aim of this is to provide a flexible, client-centred approach to care. Staff shortages and sick leave force midwives to prioritise their workload through selective visiting. Needs assessment is based on who has the greatest health need. Problems arise when the needs of all women in a given case load are comparable. One strategy commonly used to identify health need is to discuss with the client over the telephone her perceived need and that of her baby. Identification of health need in the absence of objective health criteria or comparable objective health criteria between clients is difficult. Unfortunately it is not uncommon for those who can articulate themselves well and stress the need for a visit to have their request met. This need may be prioritised above that of a client who feels less able to express her need. Studies have shown that those most in need of antenatal care are less likely to receive it. This included women who were on a low income, ethnic minority groups who had immigrated from another country of which English was not the first language, very young women and women without partners (Brown & Lumley 1993, Clement et al 1997). A study assessing satisfaction with maternity care received, found that, among 1193 postpartum women, the socially disadvantaged group were least satisfied (Brown & Lumley 1993). Other authors have discussed issues of equity in relation to antenatal home visits, where white women who owned their own homes had more of their antenatal visits at home than their black counterparts who had requested the same service (Clement et al 1997).

Exploration and acceptance of health inequalities can only serve to ensure that as far as possible midwifery supports a zero tolerance philosophy of inequality in health care provision.

Maternity services are failing women who do not fit the white middle class norm

(Bowes & Domokos 1996 pp. 45–65)

This conclusion was reached by researchers who explored the issues of empowerment and empowered ethnic minority groups within the research process. They presented findings which had not been generally voiced, many of which presented a dissonance between the needs of ethnic minority women and the provision of maternity services.

Britain became increasingly multiracial over the latter half of the twentieth century. The results of the 1996–1997 population census (Office of National Statistics 1998) state that 3.4 million people belonged to ethnic minorities in Great Britain. Despite this large representation, ethnic groups continue to experience inequalities in health care. Standards of care are jeopardised for many black and ethnic minority women who, due to communication barriers, are excluded from the privileges of empowerment and decision making and the benefits of exploring hopes and fears during antenatal education (Baxter 1993, Pearson 1985). Subsequently their choices are limited to the availability and quality of bilingual workers. The voices of many ethnic minority groups are silenced by a society which continues to marginalise and oppress them. The introduction of link workers, interpreters and advocates was a clear attempt to address the inequalities in health for maternity service users from the black and ethnic minority groups. Hackney Community Health Council (London) pioneered the first of this work in 1980. Due to the high level of Asian perinatal and infant mortality, as well as restricted access to services, the DOH launched the Asian Mother and Baby Campaign in 1984. The evaluation of the scheme demonstrated successful results, reporting high levels of consumer satisfaction and an increase in the quality of services offered to this section of the population. Other schemes have demonstrated the benefits of bilingual and advocacy workers including research commissioned by the Maternity Alliance and the Mori Health Research Unit evaluation. Reports of a reduction in antenatal admissions, antenatal stay and caesarean sections after the introduction of the bilingual health advocacy scheme, reported by an East London study (Parsons & Day 1992), is encouraging. Although other factors may have influenced these changes, the benefits to be gained from increased levels of communication should not be underestimated. The Changing Childbirth report clearly recommends that link workers and advocates should be an integral part of the maternity team and not seen as optional extras (DOH 1993). This was further endorsed by the Commission for Racial Equality's (CRE) code of conduct for maternity services (1994).

Communities with a significant ethnic minority population provide services for non-English-speaking women who use the maternity services. What happens in those areas where there are only small pockets of non-English-speaking maternity service users, or users to whom English is not their first language? It is not uncommon for family members to be used to interpret health care advice and treatment. This practice is unethical and unsafe as it leaves room for misunderstanding and clearly contravenes the Race relations code of practice in maternity services (CRE 1994).

Bridging the gap

Although race and culture form part of the curriculum for student midwifery training, racial awareness should form part of continuing education for qualified midwives. This forum should be used to heighten awareness, clarify misconceptions and enhance understanding of culture and ethnicity. As Neile (1997) suggests, experts should be utilised more during training and update sessions. Users of maternity services should also be encouraged to share their experiences at such forums. Training should not be rigidly geared toward teaching facts about ethnic groups as this approach encourages generalisations and assumptions to be made by health professionals (Schott & Henley 1996). These may include, for example, the belief that Asians have a large extended family to look after them when they get home from having their babies, therefore the support needed postnatally will be minimal. Developing policies and guidelines which are specific to certain ethnic groups in an attempt to reduce inequalities seeks to marginalise ethnic minority issues. The absence of specific consideration of ethnic minority issues may, conversely, cause the unintentional favouring of policies which benefit the ethnic majority. It is suggested that ethnic minority groups are represented appropriately on advisory bodies (Acheson 1998). Indeed support groups including the Natural Childbirth Trust could increase its membership of black and minority groups by presenting a more culturally sensitive approach to their classes which at present attract a predominantly white middle class group.

Social justice

Strategies to ensure that all members of society have an equal right to health and health care may seem utopian, but continued efforts toward meeting this standard should be adopted and remain high on the agenda of health professionals. An individual's health status is to some extent predetermined genetically. Advances in medical research have increased the likelihood of controlling some aspects of ill health, through genetic engineering. New advances in health care and screening are more accessible to the affluent members of society due to their financial capacity to access private health care. The socioeconomically disadvantaged groups should be given equal access and afforded the same privileges within the National Health Service. Improvements in environmental health, in the early part of the twentieth century, introduced environmental reforms including slum clearance, improved sanitation and clean air, which improved the population's health. Despite this major improvement, environmental factors still affect those members of society who are socioeconomically disadvantaged. People continue to live in overcrowded, damp accommodation which affects their health (Acheson 1998).

It is evident that at local level we cannot reduce inequalities in health in its entirety, but we must ensure that what we can do is effective. Social justice for users of maternity services has already been identified earlier in this chapter as being inconsistent. Consistency in the provision of health care will help to promote an equitable service. Consistency should therefore be based on criteria which is seen to be morally right. An example of this is demonstrated using the subject of pain relief. Everyone has the right to be offered the range of pain relief available, everyone has the right to have good quality, competent dialogue with a midwife exploring the advantages and disadvantages of each method, regardless of social class, ethnic orientation or language barriers. By denying this basic requirement to some users of maternity services because of judgements made about their level of intelligence or their ability to understand English, health professionals offer a second class service towards those whom society treats as second class citizens.

Health care providers purport to provide an equitable service. Value judgements can determine equity since equity is based on need within the context of the health service (Seedhouse 1988). Midwives should be vigilant when utilising needs assessment strategies for prioritising their work load. In a hospital bay, for example, where all women have had a caesarean section, the midwife can prioritise work activities according to objective criteria such as observing and recording vital signs. This can be contrasted to work in the community where the midwife is presented with a challenge of supporting clients who have psychosocial needs. Articulation of need is difficult for some women, whereas for others this does not pose as a problem. Consequently clients who are able to articulate their needs are more likely to remain satisfied with the service they receive. Midwives face challenging dilemmas in ensuring that all members of their caseload receive an equitable service.

Reflection and discussion with colleagues are useful when deciding which course of action is the most appropriate; even then it is difficult to always ensure social justice. All too often on busy labour wards midwives are set up to fail this basic requirement of service delivery. For example, when one midwife has already supported three women in labour and delivered their babies and is allocated a fourth woman during one shift can an equitable service be provided? Financial commitment to address staff shortages, support from colleagues and a critical review of personal attitudes toward the provision of health care may enable midwives to provide consistency based on what is perceived to be morally right. The implementation of clinical governance should ensure a top-down commitment toward supporting social justice. The Acheson report (1998) states that routine information systems are needed to alert clinicians and managers to changing patterns of access to health care and health outcome. The report details several recommendations which include:

- extending the focus of clinical governance to give equal prominence to equity of access to effective health care (p. 115)
- health authorities working with primary care groups and providers on local clinical governance, agreeing priorities and objectives for reducing inequalities in access to effective care; these should form part of the health improvement programme (p. 115).

Summary

- Different definitions and ideas about health may challenge health promoters' overall approach to their work.
- Health promotion planning and process will be effective and efficient if there is an understanding of health and its multiple meanings.
- Understanding the meaning of health and its broad interpretations enables an effective and efficient approach to health promotion work.
- Personal constructs of health and illness vary between individuals and cultures. Initiatives which aim to promote physical well being to the exclusion of mental and social facets of health may therefore prove ineffective.

- Health as an holistic concept refers to all dimensions of health which include: physical, mental, emotional, societal, sexual and spiritual aspects.
- Inequalities in health are still evident today; social and economic disadvantage results in the poorer members of society remaining in poor housing, experiencing unemployment and suffering from stress.
- The government document Our healthier nation (Secretary of State for Health 1999) proposes to reduce inequalities.
- Midwives contribute to the health of the nation and have an important contribution to make to women's health.
- Studies have shown that those most in need of antenatal care are less likely to receive it. This included women who were on a low income, ethnic minority groups who had immigrated from another country of which English was not the first language, very young women and women without partners.
- Babies of women in disadvantaged groups are more likely to have suffered from intrauterine growth retardation.
- Babies of fathers who are in disadvantaged groups have birth weights of 130 g lower than babies of fathers who are socioeconomically advantaged.
- There are 3.4 million people belonging to ethnic minorities in Great Britain. Despite this large representation, ethnic groups continue to experience inequalities in health care.
- Racial awareness should form part of continuing education for qualified midwives. This forum should be used to heighten the awareness and maintain the momentum of eradicating racism within all maternity services and support groups.

References

Acheson D 1998 Independent inquiry into inequalities in health. The Stationery Office, London

Barker D 1998 Mothers, babies and health in later life. Churchill Livingstone, New York

Baxter C 1993 The communication needs of black and ethnic minority women in Salford (unpublished report available from the Changing Childbirth Implementation Team)

Black D, Morris J N, Smith C, Townsend P 1982 Inequalities in health: the Black report. Penguin, Harmondsworth (first published by the DHSS, 1980. New introduction by P Townsend and N Davidson)

Blaxter M, Patterson L 1982 Mothers and daughters: a three generation study of health attitudes and behaviour. Heinemann, London

Bowes A M, Domokos T M 1996 Pakistani women and maternity care: raising muted voices. Sociology of Health and Illness 18(1):45–65

Brown S, Lumley J 1993 Antenatal care: a case of the inverse law? Australian Journal of Public Health 17:95–103

Clement S, Sikorski J, Wilson J, Das S 1997 Planning antenatal services to meet women's psychological needs. British Journal of Midwifery 5(5)

Commission For Racial Equality (CRE) 1994 Race relations code of practice in maternity services. CRE, London

Department of Health (DOH) 1992 The health of the nation targeting practice: the contribution of nurses, midwives and health visitors. DOH, London

Department of Health (DOH) 1993 Changing childbirth, part 1. Report of the Expert Maternity Group. HMSO, London

Department of Health (DOH) England, DOH Welsh Office, Scottish DOH, DOH and Social Service, Northern Ireland 1998 Why mothers die, report on the confidential enquiries into maternal deaths in the united kingdom. The Stationery Office, London

Department of Health and Social Security and Welsh Office Central Health Services Council, Standing Maternity and Midwifery Advisory Committee 1970 Domiciliary midwifery and maternity bed needs, (Peel) report of a sub-committee. HMSO, London

Dobson B, Beardsworth A, Keil T, Walker R 1994 Diet choice and poverty: social, cultural and nutritional aspects of food consumption among low income families. Loughborough University of Technology, Centre for Research in Social Policy, Loughborough

Dovey S, Bartley M, Blane D 1990 The Black report on socio-economic inequalities in health 10 years on. British Medical Journal 281:1003

Dowler E, Calvert C 1995 Nutrition and diet in lone-parent families in London. Family Policy Studies Centre, London

Downie R S, Tannahill C, Tannahill A 1996 Health promotion models and values. Oxford University Press, New York

Ellerman S 1998 Breast cancer, cultural barriers prevent effective care. Nurse Health Week, www.nurseweek.com/features/98–10/mammo.html

Ewles L, Simnett I 1999 Promoting health, a practical guide, 4th edn. Baillière Tindall, London

Gillies P, Spray J 1997 Addressing health inequalities: the practical potential of social capital. Health Education Authority, London

Graham H, Oakley A 1986 Competing ideologies of reproduction: medical and maternal perspectives on pregnancy. In: Curer C, Stacey M (eds) Concepts of health, illness and disease. Berg, Hamburg, pp 95–115

Horton R 1998 Our healthier nation possibly. The Lancet, 351 (14 February):76–77

Maslow A 1954 Motivation and personality, 2nd edn. Harper & Row, New York

Middle C, Johnson A, Alderdice F, Petty T, Macfarlane A 1996 Birth weight and health and development at seven years. Childcare, Health and Development 22:55–71

Naidoo J, Wills J 1998 Practising health promotion. Dilemmas and challenges. Baillière Tindall, London

Neile E E 1997 What midwives need to learn about race and culture. Midir's Midwifery Digest 7(1):29–33

Office for National Statistics 1998 Social Trends 28. The Stationery Office, London

Parsons L, Day S 1992 Improving obstetric outcomes in ethnic minorities: an evaluation of health advocacy in Hackney. Journal of Public Health Medicine 14(2):183–191

Pearson M 1985 Racial equality and good practice in maternity care. Training in Race and Health, London

Report of the Maternity Services Committee (Cranbrook) 1959. HMSO, London

Research Unit in Health and Behavioural Change 1989 Changing the public health. Wiley, Chichester

Royal College of Midwives (RCM) 1997 Delivery no 23. RCM, London

Safe Motherhood 1996 Adolescent health investing in the future, a newsletter of worldwide activity. World Health Organization, Geneva

Salih S 1985 Syrian poem, a woman's notebook. Exley Publications, Waford, Herts

Schott J, Henley A 1996 Culture, religion and childbearing. A handbook for professionals. Butterworth-Heinemann, London

Secretary of State for Health 1999 Our healthier nation, saving lives. The Stationery Office, London

Seedhouse D 1986 Health: foundations for achievement. John Wiley, London

Seedhouse D 1988 Ethics: the heart of health care. John Wiley, Chichester

Sutherland V, Cooper C 1990 Understanding stress. Chapman & Hall, London

Thompson A 1996 If midwives are going to contribute to the reduction of maternal mortality they have to be political as well as practice midwifery (editorial). Midwifery 12:107–108

Townsend P, Davidson N, Whitehead M (eds) 1992 Inequalities in health. Penguin, Harmondsworth

Vit T, Vatten L, Markestad T, Ahlsten G, Jacobsen G, Bakketeig L 1996 Morbidity during the first year of life in small for gestational age infants. Archives of Disease in Childhood 75:F33–F37

Whitehead M 1988 The health divide. Inequalities in health. Penguin, Harmondsworth

World Health Organization (WHO) 1946 Constitution. WHO, New York

World Health Organization (WHO) 1997 European policy for health for all. WHO Regional Office for Europe, Geneva

Recommended reading

Bright J 1997 Health promotion in clinical practice. Baillière Tindall, London

Christiani K 1996 Women's health – effect on morbidity and mortality in pregnancy and health. Midwifery 11(3):113–119

Crook S, Pakulski J, Waters M 1992 Postmodernisation: change in advanced society. Sage, London

Schott J, Henley A 1996 Culture, religion and childbearing. A handbook for professionals. Butterworth-Heinemann, London

Exploration of culture, religion and childbirth enables a critical review of personal concepts and offers clarity and new meaning to individualised approaches to health care and childbirth.

Secretary of State for Health 1998 Our healthier nation, a contract for health. A consultation paper. The Stationery Office, London

This document outlines a proposal for achieving health for all through the collaborative work of government agencies, local health authorities, local communities and health workers. The proposed contract for health provides the reader with the government's intention for improving health in the twenty-first century.

Seedhouse D 1986 Health: foundations for achievement. John Wiley, London

This text offers the reader an opportunity to explore personal ideas of health and presents a philosophical approach to health and health for all.

2

Health promotion – models and values, an integral part of midwifery practice

Key themes

- What is health promotion?
- Antenatal health education, the cornerstone of health promotion in midwifery
- Assessing health needs
- Different approaches to health promotion: medical, behaviour change, educational, client centred, societal change, self-empowerment
- Informed health choices, fact or fiction?
- Models of health promotion
- Social capital and the midwife
- Ethics and health promotion

Overview

This chapter explores the meaning of 'health promotion' and its application to midwifery practice. Several approaches and models to health promotion are highlighted, demonstrating the scope of health promotion work. The notion of empowerment is critiqued in detail, as an important approach to health promotion work. Ideas about choice and control are challenged within the context of health promotion and midwifery. The chapter continues with the philosophy of health defined in Chapter 1 and relates this critically to the approaches of health promotion explored.

What is health promotion?

Health promotion has become increasingly fashionable since the 1980s. The concept was first used in the 1970s by the Canadian Minister of National Health and Welfare, Marc Lalonde. This perspective on health promotion identified determinants of health by environment and individual behaviours and lifestyles, not by biomedical characteristics. This influenced further ideas on the definition of health promotion. The World Health Organization in future years changed the emphasis of health promotion from medical care to primary health care, which was reflected in global policy. The 1977 World Health Assembly at Alma Ata consigned all member countries to raise the standards of health and reduce inequalities in health to a standard which assured all people of productive lives (World Health Organization 1986). Today health promotion is interpreted and used in a number of different ways. It may be described as a process by which individuals or groups are encouraged to adopt healthy lifestyles, the focus of which is behavioural change. Other ideas include: preventing ill health, maintaining positive health, raising public awareness of health issues, protecting the public from harm, educating people to make healthy lifestyle choices and reducing inequalities in health and the provision of health care. Health promotion may be viewed as:

- a sale of goods, where health is a commodity easily acquired
- glamorous one-off campaign which seeks to reassure those out of touch with reality that they make a difference to inequality.

It is fair to surmise that the multiplicity of meanings and ideas of health promotion reduce its ability to be recognised as a discipline. Activities which seek to improve health are often labelled as 'health promotion work'. Yeo (1993) views health promotion as any intervention aimed at enabling people to enhance their health. It is suggested, however, that broad definitions of health promotion render the process meaningless and open to wide interpretation (Downie, Tannahill & Tannahill 1996). WHO defines health promotion as: 'The process of enabling people to increase control over their health, and improve it' (WHO 1984). Integral to the definition is the notion of empowerment and the reduction of professional dominance. However, socioeconomic and cultural differences involved in the enabling process are not acknowledged. Tones (1992) suggests that health promotion should seek to ensure the most efficient delivery of health and medical services. It should facilitate choice of a health lifestyle and create a physical and socioeconomic environment which fosters health and reduces the likelihood of illness.

Recognising that health promotion had acquired so many different meanings, Tannahill (1985) developed a model of health promotion which provides a framework for the range of activities integral to health promotion work (see Fig. 2.2). The results of this study shaped the following definition: 'Health promotion comprises efforts to enhance positive health and reduce the risk of ill-health, through overlapping spheres of health education, prevention, and health protection' (Downie, Tannahill & Tannahill 1996 p. 60). The definition limits the scope of health promotion to three fundamental areas and leaves little room for speculation of its meaning. It is, however, difficult to define health promotion in its entirety, and parallels may be drawn with the dilemmas highlighted in Chapter 1 when attempting to define health.

Health promotion and health education

It is not uncommon for health promotion to be confused with health education. The terms should not be used interchangeably. Health promotion covers all aspects of activities which seek to promote healthy lifestyles; health education is an integral part of this process. Dines & Crib (1993) describe health promotion as a wider-ranging term than health education and refer to it as 'health education plus'. This description provides little clarity for the scope of health promotion work. Health promotion activities which involve, for example, community development work and political action go far beyond the scope of health education and are encompassed in the broader discipline of health promotion. The traditional approach to health education was aimed at preventing ill health, as opposed to enhancing positive health. The origins of this approach lie in the nineteenth century when people were lectured and scaremongered into leading healthy lifestyles to prevent disease. The focus of modern health education is working with the individual toward a stage or state of health through enabling strategies. It uses a broad information base and educational principles which are facilitative. This approach recognises that cajoling and scaremongering are counterproductive to maintaining and achieving health. The cornerstone of modern health education is empowerment (Tones 1992). Modern health education is seen as an important element of health promotion. The midwife is actively involved in both health promotion and health education and has a unique relationship with the woman and her family to influence the adoption of a healthy lifestyle (see Box 2.1).

Scope for midwifery practice – health promotion, health protection and ill health prevention

Some examples of the scope of health promotion in midwifery are listed in Box 2.1. (Other examples of health protection, ill health prevention and health education are highlighted later in the chapter.)

Health needs

Assessing health need enables the identification of target areas for health promotion work. The clients' health needs are varied and are perceived as

Box 2.1 **Examples of health promotion in midwifery**

- Reducing the prevalence of smoking during pregnancy is considered health promotion. Health education is integral to this process.
- Discussing postnatal depression during pregnancy is health promotion, involving health education and health protection.
- Ensuring that a mother is given an injection of anti-D immunoglobulin is health promotion involving prevention of ill health and health protection.
- Teaching parenting skills is health promotion involving health education, health protection and ill health prevention.
- Raising awareness of safe limits of alcohol ingestion during pregnancy is health promotion, involving health protection and ill health prevention and health education.
- Discussing the benefits of exercise is health promotion, involving health education.

need based on subjective criteria. This means that the midwife's perception of health need may differ from that of the client. The manager's criteria for health need may differ from that of the midwife. Naidoo & Wills (1998) suggest that the purpose of need must be justifiable for it to be perceived as a need. Ewles & Simnett (1999) state that the ideal situation in which to determine need is a joint decision by clients and health promoters. This leaves room for resolving conflict of interests and limited scope for imposing alien values on the client.

To examine further whose needs would be considered justifiable, consider the following scenarios.

Scenario 1

Geraldine lives in a one-bedroomed flat situated within a high rise block. She is 35 weeks' pregnant and is booked to have a caesarean section for placenta praevia grade IV. Geraldine has two other children, both under 5 years old. Both children suffer from asthma. Her partner is supportive when he is around. Unfortunately he will be out of the country for the next 6 months. Geraldine has a drug and drink problem and feels that she **needs** help.

Scenario 2

Jade is a 36-year-old primigravida who has progressed well during her pregnancy and has no identified adverse risk factors. Her husband who is also her business partner is very supportive. The pregnancy was timed carefully so that the delivery did not interfere with business plans. Unfortunately, however, Jade needed to deliver at 38 weeks' gestation in order to fulfil a major opportunistic business venture. Her husband couldn't fulfil this requirement. She desperately **needed** to have caesarean section and expressed her need to her consultant.

Scenario 3

Ben has been a midwife for 8 years, he has a keen interest in antenatal education and is responsible for resources. He teaches antenatal education within his group practice and facilitates postnatal groups. The women and their families who attended his classes have complained about the chairs and find it difficult to sit, rise and stay sitting for even short periods. The floor is unsuitable for sitting and there are no bean bags. He has expressed a **need** for comfortable chairs to be purchased for the past 3 years.

Scenario 4

The head of midwifery services recognises a **need** to increase the number of perineal repair workshops for midwives. Eighty per cent of midwives within the maternity unit are capable of perineal repair, but only 40% use the technique, which has been shown through current research-based evidence to reduce perineal morbidity.

Scenario 5

The catchment area for maternity unit 'A' has a large proportion of ethnic groups who do not speak English, and book for maternity care. Fortunately the unit is well staffed with support workers, many of whom are multilingual and meet the needs of the cultural group attending. Six miles away, maternity unit 'B' also has a large proportion of ethnic groups who book for maternity care and do not speak English. Unfortunately they do not employ link workers and so the midwives and the women try to communicate with each other, as well as they are able. Maternity unit 'B' has a clear **need**.

Bradshaw's (1972) taxonomy of needs identifies four different types: normative, felt, expressed and comparative need.

Normative needs – for a practice example see Scenarios 3 and 4

These are determined by the professional and are objective in nature. They may be determined by, for example, a low uptake of prenatal folic acid or a decrease in successful breast-feeding rates. Identified needs are based on objective criteria including performance indicators and policy recommendations. Once the need is identified, an appropriate health promotion strategy to address it is determined. Evaluation would be an essential part of this process (see Ch. 11).

Felt needs – for a practice example see Scenario 1

These are determined by the individual. They are an expression of the individual's true personal need. Personal health needs may be culturally determined by criteria of health and ill health. Due to their subjective nature they are likely to be viewed critically by others. It is not uncommon to remain in the felt need taxonomy for a considerable length of time.

Expressed needs – for a practice example see Scenario 2

This is concerned with expressing a felt need, where the client asks for help. It cannot be assumed, however, that all individuals are able to express their need. This is greatly influenced by: how the individuals perceive the health professionals to whom the need is expressed, whether individuals feel they have a right to express their need and if they are able to articulate their need. Ultimately the nature of how a need is expressed is determined by individual social and cultural influences. Individuals who pay for private health care may believe that they have a right to express their need. There is a tendency to listen to those who shout the loudest or those who appear to have the greater influence.

Comparative needs – for a practice example see Scenario 5

The situation where people do not have the same service provision as those with similar needs is referred to as comparative need. Addressing comparative need inevitably helps to reduce inequalities in health and health care provision.

It is clear that health needs are anything but straightforward. When government policy reflects a health need as priority above another area considered by its constituency to be of greater need, issues of moral and ethical conflict may be apparent. One could argue that all needs are justifiable. The health service may perceive justifiable health needs in terms of cost effectiveness with regards to health gain and the end justifying the means. The maternity services determine health need by, for example, the results of maternity service satisfaction surveys, assessment of local population needs, data regarding morbidity, mortality, smoking cessation rates, breast-feeding rates and the incidence of teenage pregnancies. Evaluation and audit are also useful mechanisms for determining health need.

The aim of health promotion

Establishing a clear aim for health promotion activities provides focus and intent for the development and progression of health promotion programmes. A common aim for health promoters is to change individual behaviour and lifestyles; some may also seek to improve social support, develop community health improvement programmes and empower members of the community to take control over their health behaviour. Concentration on the former presents only a limited approach and does not acknowledge socioeconomic disadvantage, poverty and oppression as factors which influence lifestyle and behaviour traits. Attention only to the latter does not encourage individualised approaches to health promotion, for example intensive counselling and personal skills development, which have been shown to encourage health-related behaviour change in one in four of those who participate (Gillies & Spray 1997).

The aim of the health promotion initiative will ultimately determine the approach taken (see Table 2.1).

Different approaches to health promotion

The approach used by health professionals can have a positive or negative effect on the subsequent individual's behaviour. The approach chosen is largely determined by personal interpretation and understanding of health and health promotion, explored so far. There are in excess of 90 approaches and models in health promotion, some of which are better known than others (Rawson 1992). Tones (1992) identified four approaches to promoting health: the self-empowerment approach, which seeks to increase self-esteem and encourage decision-making skills, the educational approach, which seeks to empower people to make informed choices, the preventative approach, which seeks to change behaviours which may cause disease, and the radical approach, which involves identifying socioeconomic and political factors which affect health. Similarly, Ewles & Simnett (1999) identify five approaches to health promotion: the medical or preventative approach, behavioural change, educational, client-centred and societal change approaches. Understanding the significance of health promotion approaches will highlight the benefits of one approach complementing the other.

The medical approach

This approach is conceptualised around the absence of disease. It seeks to prevent ill health and premature death through medical intervention. The medical approach has its roots in preventative medicine. Successful results have been demonstrated in public health, with immunisation and vaccination programmes minimising childhood disease. It does, however, encourage medical dependency for knowledge and relies on persuasive tactics to ensure compliance. Prevention and cure are priority areas to the exclusion of socio-economic disadvantage as a cause of ill health. Activities to develop this approach include widespread media campaigns and education. The overall aim of the medical approach is to reduce morbidity and premature mortality. Its focus is primarily based on persuasive tactics and puts the onus of responsibility on the individual to make healthy choices to prevent disease.

The criticism of the preventative model is widely documented (Tones 1981, Vuori 1980). It embraces a victim-blaming ideology and ignores the sociocultural and political aspects of health.

The behavioural change approach

This approach is concerned with encouraging people to adopt healthy behaviours and is frequently used within health care. The approach assumes that people are free to make choices about making a health-related behavioural change. An appreciation of the socioeconomic and cultural barriers to making healthy lifestyle choices and the complex process involved in health-related behavioural change is a prerequisite to its use. Health promotion activities used for this approach include: communication and counselling, education, empowerment, decision making, fostering community groups and building social support networks. Although the focus for evaluation is clear when using this approach, problems may be evident as some people take longer to change than others.

The educational approach

This approach is concerned with facilitating the learning process and enabling learning to take place through open dialogue and discussion. Valuing life experiences and tailoring education to meet individual needs are integral to this process. (This is explored further in Ch. 10.) To raise awareness and begin the process of education mass media campaigns have been used with varying degrees of success.

However, mass media campaigns reach only those members of the population who have a motivation towards change. They may also be counterproductive. Using media tactics the Health Education Authority (HEA, poster presentation, 1992) sought to raise awareness of the risks associated with smoking during pregnancy. This involved the illustration of a neonate in an incubator, with a nasogastric tube down its nose. A large bold caption, stated, at the bottom of the poster, **'For the last nine months he's been smoking cigarettes, now he's on to a pipe'** (and in smaller non-descript print) 'giving up smoking is not easy, especially when you're pregnant. If you'd like some sympathetic advice call the quit line on 071–487 3000'. The aim of the campaign was to raise awareness about the harmful effects of tobacco during pregnancy and motivate women toward behaviour change. Instead, however, it may increase feelings of guilt and stress, which may be relieved by the aid of another cigarette. The onus of responsibility lies with the individual. The effectiveness and efficiency of mass media campaigns have caused concern (Flay et al 1993). It is difficult to measure the different ways they influence and motivate people toward changing their health behaviour. The negative consequences are equally difficult to measure.

The client-centred approach

This approach is based on an equal partnership between the health

Reflection points

- Which health promotion approach have you used during clinical practice?

- What factors determined the approach used?

- How do you determine the success of the approach used?

Reflection point

- Reflect on how you facilitate the process of decision making with clients. Which factors may have influenced the decision-making process, firstly from the client's perspective and then from the professional's perspective?

professional and the client. The agenda is set by the client and the health professional's role is facilitative – guiding, supporting and encouraging the client to make informed choices. The aim is concerned with facilitating client autonomy.

The societal change approach

The aim of this approach is to ensure that health is easier to achieve and supports the notion of 'health for all'. The focus is not on changing individual behaviour, but on positively influencing the health of society.

This approach acknowledges socioeconomic disadvantage as a determinant of ill health. It is concerned with making environmental, social and economic changes by policy planning, political action and widespread collaboration with decision makers.

Midwifery practice – approaches to health promotion

There is not one 'right' approach or set of activities for health promotion. Table 2.1 illustrates the varied scope of health promotion in midwifery practice and the approach utilised for health promotion.

Self-empowerment approach

The process of self-empowerment involves people identifying their personal concerns, strengths, experiences and skills and utilising them to increase control over their own lives. Increasing self-awareness and improving self-esteem are an integral part of this process. The health promoter acts as a facilitator by offering support and guidance. Tones (1992) suggests that self-empowerment focuses on individuals' capacity to take control over their own lives. Bright (1997) offers strategies to ensure that self-empowerment is possible. They include helping people to develop personal skills and self-esteem and the provision of accurate information and knowledgeable, appropriate advice.

It is a fallacy to believe that all adults in society are autonomous. Autonomy is a state that is acquired but is not attainable by all people. A proposal put forward by Downie, Tannahill & Tannahill (1996) suggests reasons why. In an attempt to make right a person's ill health, medical experts with an overzealous curative nature have conveyed a strong message that an individual cannot manage his or her own health. It is suggested that this has happened insidiously over a number of years (Downie, Tannahill & Tannahill 1996). The medicalisation of an experience has attributed to the need to seek outside help, prior to exploring personal resources. People have therefore lost confidence in their own ability to take control.

Health concern	Health promotion initiative	Health promotion approach	Health promotion activity	
Breast-feeding rates below the national average	• Raise awareness about the benefits of breast feeding, enabling those women who wish to breast feed to do so successfully • Support women who are unsure of their feeding intention toward making informed decisions	• Client-centred approach	• One to one work may include: – exploration of values, attitudes, and breast-feeding influences; – discussion, education, one to one midwife to client support facilitation; – feeding intention	**Table 2.1** **The scope of health promotion in midwifery practice**
		• Educational approach	• Breast-feeding workshops may include: – information, knowledge, discussion, reflection, empowerment; – development of decision-making skills	
		• Societal change approach	• Political/community action toward a breast-feeding friendly environment	
		• Behavioural change approach	• Workshops may include: – exploration and discussion; – establish whether the client is precontemplating, contemplating, or ready for action, apply the appropriate strategy to meet the client's assessed current position	

	Health concern	Health promotion initiative	Health promotion approach	Health promotion activity
Table 2.1 (cont'd)	• One-third of pregnant women who book for maternity care and smoke continue to do so throughout the remainder of the pregnancy	• Raise awareness of the effects of cigarette smoke on the woman, fetus and family members, enabling those women who wish to give up to do so successfully • Raise awareness of the benefits of cessation	• Client-centred approach	• One to one work may include: – exploration of values and attitudes; – exploration of reasons why smoking continues; – discussion on the nature of the smoking behaviour • One to one continued support • Inclusion of family members who smoke • Facilitation of informed choices
			• Educational approach	• Workshops may include: – information, knowledge, discussion • Development of skills • Exploration of strategies for stopping, staying stopped and maintenance of non-smoking behaviour • Information and discussion re: damage limitation strategies for women who wish to continue (see Ch. 6) • Family education

Table 2.1
(cont'd)

Health concern	Health promotion initiative	Health promotion approach	Health promotion activity
		• Societal change approach	• Political/social action toward adopting smoke free zones
		• Behavioural change approach	• Workshops may include: – exploration of client's position on the behavioural change cycle (precontemplator, contemplator, ready for action) • Apply appropriate health promotion intervention • Self-empowerment • Involve family members • Support decision, continuity of carer one to one support, community support, i.e. stop-smoking groups, quit line information
Only 5% of antenatal and postnatal women perform pelvic floor exercises	• Raise awareness of the benefits of pelvic floor exercises	• Client-centred approach	• One to one work may include: – exploration of values and attitudes; – discussion on the benefits of pelvic floor exercises; – exploration of strategies to ensure compliance, self-empowerment

	Health concern	Health promotion initiative	Health promotion approach	Health promotion activity
Table 2.1 *(cont'd)*			• Educational approach	• Information, knowledge, discussion • Development of skills, practice to ensure competence (see Ch. 8) • Explore stategies which will ensure maintenance • Continued education, support, continuity to encourage maintenance, self-empowerment

Enabling people to take control is not as simple as saying, for example, 'it's up to you to make a choice', or 'it's your responsibility'. This approach directs total responsibility toward the client and assumes understanding, accurate interpretation and an ability to make inferences about the information received. If a choice is made based on this premise and the outcome is adverse then the burden of guilt is encumbered on the person who made the choice. Making the right decision is a difficult process particularly for women who are consumers of maternity services. Individuals may require help and support with regards to resources, know-how and power in order to assume greater control when making decisions. It is suggested, therefore, that the process of enabling should be nurtured and developed and not assumed (Yeo 1993).

Individuals' capacity to take control over their lives is the central theme of self-empowerment. For instance, consider environmental circumstances, which may either facilitate the exercise of control or present a barrier to free action. The hospital may present a barrier for women who choose to attend antenatal education classes. Midwives work hard to make the environment for their classes as informal and relaxed as possible and attempt to reduce barriers to participation by facilitating the process of positive group dynamics (Ch. 10 explores the benefits of group dynamics further). Taylor (1979) noted that the hospital was one of the few places where individuals forfeit control over virtually every task they customarily perform. Nearly two decades later traits of this are still apparent. The birth plan was a concerted effort to enable clients to exert some control over childbirth. The aim of the birth plan is to give clients the opportunity to make decisions about childbirth, giving them a sense of control and encouraging the philosophy of a partnership approach to care. By exploration and discussion of choices available, birth plans are completed. The ethical importance of the principles of autonomy are stressed, which leaves little room for the imposition of foreign values.

The extent to which individuals believe that they are in control deserves consideration. There is a clear demarcation between individuals who believe they are in control and those who possess the necessary skills and competencies to influence what happens to them. Lewis (1986) sheds interesting light on different varieties of control. Reference is made to a type of control which involves discussion with clients, but does not allow them any chance of influencing the decision made. This is referred to as 'processual control'. It can be argued that such tokenism can be beneficial to clients as they have an illusionary belief that they have influenced the decision by merely having a discussion. This is further supported by Langer (1983), who suggests that even the illusion of control is acceptable. Feelings of control are generally accompanied by emotional feelings of self-worth and self-esteem. It has generally been assumed that a sense of control is associated with a good level of self-esteem. Those who have a high level of self-esteem are probably less likely to accept and tolerate the dissonance of knowingly engaging in a behaviour that is injurious to health. They are therefore more likely to do something about it as opposed to an individual who has a low self-esteem (Tones 1992). Curie & Todd (1992) challenged this notion when observing self-esteem in teenage boys who smoked; smoking among 15–16-year-old males was found to be more common in those with high self-esteem. A possible explanation, however, is that a high level of self-esteem is partially due to smoking. Generally a high self-esteem contributes to true well being and feelings of self-worth.

Reflection points

- Reflect on the opportunities for making choices from the moment clients find out they are pregnant.

- Are all clients afforded the same opportunities to make choices?

- Is it possible to provide clients with appropriate information to enable them to exercise control over the choices they make?

- How much control do clients have?

- What factors determine client control?

Now you can make your choice

Health promotion work is involved with empowering people to make healthy lifestyle choices. This may involve work specifically targeted toward behavioural change, or raising awareness about strategies for attaining and/or maintaining positive health. Despite the provision of current research-based evidence and empowering clients to make choices, the freedom to choose a healthier lifestyle is very often limited. Women may be well informed, but can they truly make healthy lifestyle choices? People live their lives in different social contexts each relating to cultural or group norms. Circumstances within such contexts influence the individual's freedom of choice. Choice may be confounded by:

- addiction to, for example, nicotine
- economic factors which inhibit the intake of a healthy diet
- lack of social support
- poverty and social deprivation
- professional bias.

As previously mentioned, individuals may require help and support with regards to resources, know-how and power, in order to assume greater control when making decisions.

Consider the case study in Box 2.2. Socioeconomic circumstances limit Tina's choices. Cigarettes are used as a coping strategy. Making a lifestyle change requires planning, focus and commitment in order to be successful. Stressful circumstances which include bereavement, poverty, abuse and lack of support are challenging and stressful, even without the attempt to change the one behaviour which provides temporary relief. Economically it could be argued that Tina has the freedom to choose between a potentially health-destroying behaviour and a presumably healthy diet. Tina feels that smoking helps her psychological well being and reduces stress levels. It is suggested that, in situations where such circumstances exist, health choices

Box 2.2 **Case study: Tina**

The following study demonstrates how the health professional intends the client to be able to make an informed choice, but the client's perception at the end of the interaction is that there is no choice.

Tina is a 28-year-old unemployed woman who is expecting her fifth baby. She has four children under the age of 7 years and is a single parent. Tina lives in a two-bedroomed small flat with her new partner and his 11-year-old son. Her partner is abusive toward her and spends the majority of her social support money on alcohol. Tina informs the midwife that this leaves her in a difficult position to buy and eat a healthy diet. Tina smokes 20 cigarettes per day and considers her 'smoke' to be the only thing that helps her to cope with life. She has recently lost her mother from lung cancer. Tina would like to give up smoking during her pregnancy. She informs the midwife that three of her children have asthma and she thinks that it is due to her smoking. She feels guilty about this, which causes her stress and causes her to smoke more. She is counselled about stopping smoking and is asked to set a stop date.

Tina continues to smoke, she feels that she has **no** choice.

become health compromises (Ewles & Simnett 1999). Unfortunately the healthier choice is not always the easier choice. It could be argued that Tina needs to change her social circumstances which are potentially health debilitating. The situation then leads to victim blaming, which is counter-productive, encourages feelings of guilt and ultimately reinforces the need to smoke. The following areas proposed by Tones (1991) highlight factors which may influence the level of control people have over their own lifestyles:

- environmental circumstances, which may either facilitate the exercise of control or present a barrier to free action
- the extent to which individuals actually possess competencies or skills that enable them to control some aspect of their lives and perhaps overcome environmental barriers
- the extent to which individuals believe they are in control
- various states or traits that typically accompany different beliefs about control, for example feelings of helplessness, depression and lack of self-worth.

Limitation of screening programmes by health agencies is one example of how choices about healthier lifestyles are inhibited. Reduced availability of screening services limits the opportunity to make informed choices about potential health risks. A current example is the availability of human immunodeficiency virus (HIV) screening for pregnant women. In 1992 the DOH recommended that all women should be offered HIV screening in areas of high prevalence, and women considered to be high risk offered screening in areas with low prevalence. The Unlinked Anonymous Surveys Steering Group (1997) found that for every five pregnant women with HIV only one knew her HIV status before the birth of the baby. Therefore only one women was given the opportunity to make choices about drug treatment, delivery and postpartum management to reduce the risk of vertical transmission to her fetus. Routine offering of HIV testing for pregnant women provides an opportunity for women to make choices about establishing their HIV status and therefore exert greater control over their health and that of their baby. (Ch. 5 explores this in further detail.)

Self-empowerment cannot be discussed without exploring the nature of community empowerment. This involves empowering members of the community to enable them to work toward social change by challenging social and political issues (see section on social capital). This may or may not progress toward raising political consciousness.

Whichever approach is chosen to carry out health promotion work, the midwife's role is one of enabling and supporting rather than cajoling and coercing. Empowering women to make choices about adopting health behaviours can only seek to promote long term health gain.

Models of health promotion

Four perspectives of health promotion

Caplan & Holland (1990) suggest that there are four ways of looking at health promotion (Fig. 2.1), generated from two dimensions. The first dimension is concerned with theories which focus on the nature of society, which range from radical change to social regulation. Radical change is concerned with socioeconomic and political change which seeks to relieve social conflicts such as racism and subordination of certain classes and groups. Social regulation is concerned with society existing in a state of unity and order, where institutions serve to meet the needs of citizens, in an approach that fosters cultural belonging and identity. The second dimension is concerned with the nature of scientific knowledge and assumes that there is a subjective or objective approach to acquiring knowledge. How health promotion is viewed is determined by how knowledge is acquired, via either the objective or subjective approach or a combination of both. The model illustrated in Figure 2.1 brings together the theories of society and the approaches to scientific knowledge, resulting in four perspectives on health promotion. Each perspective represented within a quadrant offers an understanding of health and health promotion: the radical humanistic perspective, the radical structuralist perspective, the humanist perspective and the traditional perspective.

Figure 2.1
Four paradigms or perspectives of health promotion (after Caplan & Holland 1990, with permission of W. B. Saunders)

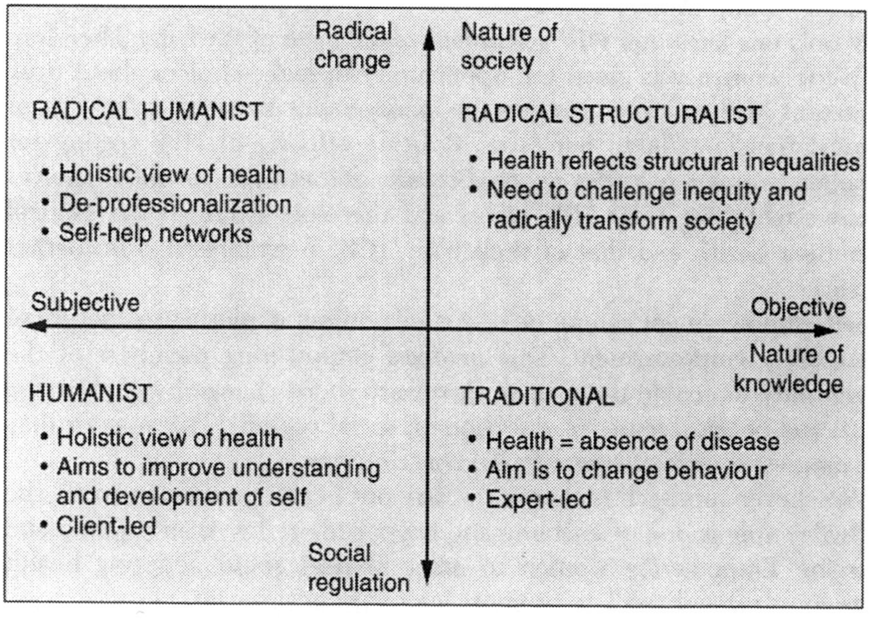

Radical change — Nature of society

RADICAL HUMANIST
- Holistic view of health
- De-professionalization
- Self-help networks

RADICAL STRUCTURALIST
- Health reflects structural inequalities
- Need to challenge inequity and radically transform society

Subjective ← → Objective

Nature of knowledge

HUMANIST
- Holistic view of health
- Aims to improve understanding and development of self
- Client-led

TRADITIONAL
- Health = absence of disease
- Aim is to change behaviour
- Expert-led

Social regulation

Radical humanist perspective

This is concerned with helping people to take and have control over their own lives. Health promotion would foster the notion of empowerment and seek, through community enlightenment, social support networks. Health is viewed from an holistic viewpoint encompassing the mind, body and spirit.

Radical structuralist perspective

This is concerned with inequalities in health, including racism and discrimination, as determinants of health. This health promotion approach would seek to challenge the fabric of society that through inequality of opportunity seeks to maintain the affluent status quo.

Humanist perspective

This is concerned with the client-centred approach of education and counselling where individuals are encouraged to identify and utilise personal strength toward health gain. Health is viewed from an holistic viewpoint.

Traditional perspective

This is concerned with the medical approach to health and health promotion. Health is viewed as the absence of disease. Behavioural change is integral to this perspective of health promotion. Professional boundaries are maintained, supporting the philosophy of medical dominance.

Each quadrant adopts a different philosophy and assumption about the nature of knowledge and society. It is suggested that to hold one approach precludes the adoption of others (Naidoo & Wills 1998). However, the humanist and radical humanist perspectives would foster similar health promotion approaches to achieve the desired aim.

> **Discussion questions**
> - Refer to Figure 2.1. Consider the four perspectives of health promotion as proposed there. Discuss with your colleagues ways in which this model could be applied to midwifery practice.
> - What are the strengths and weaknesses of the model?

Tannahill's model of health promotion

Tannahill (1985) developed a model of health promotion (Fig. 2.2) that is intended to provide a framework whereby health advocates can identify, plan and carry out health promotion. It presents health promotion as a process which has interconnected spheres of health education, prevention and health protection, ensuring that one does not exist without the other (Tannahill 1985). The different sections should not be viewed as rigidly separate from each other, however.

The model demonstrates the scope of health promotion, albeit rather descriptively. It illustrates how one approach to health promotion warrants the inclusion of another in order to be effective. Naidoo & Wills (1998) suggest that the areas of distinction and overlap can cause disagreement.

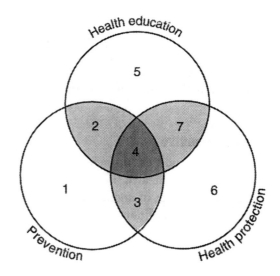

Figure 2.2
A model of health promotion (from Tannahill 1985, Health Education Journal, by permission of Oxford University Press)

Social capital and the midwife: a strategy for health promotion within primary care groups

Health promotion is said to work best for all members of society if it seeks to tackle the socioeconomic and environmental arena, in which individuals live their everyday lives. Social capital is concerned with health promotion at this level and involves the forging of partnerships which encourage, enhance and value social relationships. In its crudest sense social capital:

- fosters a culture of social support
- involves forging networks for the exchange of information
- develops a culture which encourages health-related behavioural change
- involves groups of people who create an environment of social trust through interacting with organisations and social systems to produce benefits for society and individuals in society.

Forging partnerships between the public and professional groups, sharing ideas and maximising the potential for sharing learning resources serve to facilitate community empowerment. To achieve maximum benefit from community approaches, Gillies & Spray (1997) suggest the need for volunteer work, peer programmes and civic activities, for example voting. In addition, to sustain the impact, they suggest that there is a need for policies at local and national level.

The development of groups within the community which enhance and value social relationships, act as social support systems and establish networks for information through the formation of partnerships is referred to as 'social capital' in the community setting. Its aim is concerned with healing the social ills of society and encouraging cohesive community networks. The focus of social capital is a means of collectively breaking down barriers to health care and health information and forging partnerships between health professionals and lay representatives of the community, to enable health promotion to make a substantial contribution to the poorer members of the community. The potential for the midwife's contribution to health promotion in the community is vastly underdeveloped. The ideas and recent developments, including community clinics, drop-in clinics, drop-in parentcraft, meet the midwife sessions and health promotion stalls, are potential starting points for building social resources.

Wilkinson (1996) suggests that building social capital would help to reduce the relative inequalities in society and encourage social cohesiveness. Indeed this would encourage community trust and support, but somehow it devolves the government of responsibility and puts the onus on a 'do it yourself' philosophy.

Community groups have gained momentum in establishing health gain. The 'healthy start' programme in Canada involved community partnerships which involved local people and collaboration with the health and welfare sectors. The aim was to improve health and development outcomes for children. There were noted improvements in parenting skills and uptake of food and nutritional programmes (Bhatti 1997). Good social relationships, social trust and civic activities are fundamental requirements for health outcomes (Gillies & Spray 1997). The following are suggested criteria for success (Gillies & Spray 1997):

- carrying out of a local needs assessment
- encouraging agencies to work together and maintain their commitment and contact
- representation and involvement of people from the local community
- recognition of the need for training and support for those actively involved to achieve maximum impact
- establishment of a local committee which provides the foundation for the whole process
- political access
- appropriate resource allocation
- adaptability and flexibility
- development and implementation of policies and guidelines
- cross-boundary working of professional and lay representatives.

Measuring social capital

Community initiatives which involve integrated peer support, empowerment, improved decision-making skills, feelings of social support and levels of community involvement are difficult to measure. It is suggested that these activities are considered as functionings and outputs. New social indicators should be developed to deal with new approaches in health promotion. The utilisation of the existing techniques to measure effectiveness of community or partnership approaches may underestimate their value and effectiveness (Biriotti 1997). (Ch. 11 elaborates further on evaluation techniques.)

Ethics and health promotion

Health promotion is an integral part of the midwife's role; this, however, does not exclude the midwife's work from ethical scrutiny. The nature of health promotion work in midwifery is geared toward promoting the health of the mother and ensuring an optimum environment for the fetus. The ultimate aim is to enable the safe delivery of a healthy newborn to a mother and partner who are physically and psychologically well adjusted to parenthood. The proposal of adopting a healthy lifestyle is in the interest of both the fetus and the woman. Conflict arises when the mother bears the burden of responsibility for not adopting or changing her behaviour to optimise the health environment of the fetus. It is unlikely, however, that the infant could sue the mother for not changing a behaviour such as smoking during pregnancy. The fetus is not regarded as having an independent legal personality until it is born. The Congenital Disabilities Act 1976 gives the infant the right to sue for the harm caused by negligent actions of the mother or father which resulted in the adverse condition of the infant (Dimond 1994). The midwife's position also warrants consideration, as midwives understand the implications involved for the fetus when behaviours including smoking and drinking and substance abuse continue throughout the preconception period and pregnancy. Health promotion strategies employed to encourage the adoption of healthy life choices should not be coercive and create the notion of victim blaming.

Consider the scenario in Box 2.3. Do you feel that the effects in the above scenario in terms of health gain are justifiable? Did you notice that the word 'breast' was omitted from the conversation once Jasmine had given up breast feeding. Despite verbal and non-verbal communication problems, assumptions and lack of awareness, health promotion activities in theory should affect peoples lives in an health-enhancing manner but all too often well-intentioned health promoters become potential health destroyers.

Box 2.3 **Case study: Jasmine**

Jasmine delivered her first baby 3 days ago. During the antenatal period she had decided to breast feed because she was told that it was the best food for the baby. Jasmine attended antenatal education sessions and a breast-feeding workshop. Her partner and extended family were supportive of her plans. Unfortunately Jasmine was finding breast feeding very difficult; it was not as easy as she thought. Her nipples felt sore and painful. Jasmine felt very distressed and cried when alone. She found the whole experience soul destroying. Jasmine felt that she wanted to start bottle feeding her baby, so that she could begin to enjoy the experience of motherhood without the stress of trying to breast feed. Her named midwife reassured her that things would get better and ensured that her technique was correct. She even sat with Janice throughout two feeds a day (a luxury many can ill afford). Jasmine, however, grew increasingly unhappy and felt that she did not want to continue to breast feed. Her midwife continued to offer lots of support, encouragement and reassurance as she knew how important it was that Jasmine persevere. Each time the midwife arrived to help her to feed her baby, Jasmine felt distressed, resentful toward the midwife and did not feel in control of the situation. She changed the baby to formulae feed and gave up breast feeding on her fifth postnatal day. She contacted the midwife and told her that she no longer needed her help with feeding the baby as she was now quite confident; she thanked her for her support. Jasmine never disclosed to the midwife that she had given up breast feeding. The midwife visited Jasmine on two more occasions, one of which was the discharge visit. When asked how the feeding was going, Jasmine always replied, 'fine'.

Summary

- The midwife is actively involved in both health promotion and health education and has a unique relationship with the woman and her family to influence the adoption of a healthy lifestyle.
- Health promotion interventions, including counselling, personal skills development and self-help manuals, have shown significant success in health-related behavioural change.
- It is the poorer members of society who are least likely to take part in such efforts and even if they do are less likely to succeed.
- Health promotion is more effective when it functions at a level that is within the context of people's everyday lives, acknowledging the environmental and social structures which continue to have debilitating influences on health.
- The approach used by health professionals can have a positive or negative effect on the individual's subsequent behaviour. The approach chosen is largely determined by personal interpretation and understanding of health and health promotion.

- There are in excess of 90 approaches and models in health promotion, some of which are better known than others. Approaches to promoting health include: the self-empowerment approach, which seeks to increase self-esteem and encourage decision-making skills, the educational approach, which seeks to empower people to make informed choices, the preventative approach, which seeks to change behaviours which may cause disease, and the radical approach, which involves identifying socioeconomic and political factors which affect health.
- Health promotion practice has not uniformly kept pace with advances in theory.
- Unfortunately time and resources and possibly a reduced knowledge base may encourage the employment of the traditional health education approaches. An awareness of this shortfall can be a positive start in challenging time and resource limitations at local and national level.
- Health promotion should involve encouragement for strengthening human potential.
- Health promotion strategies should be culturally sensitive to increase the chances of efficacy.
- Health education is intrinsic to health promotion; the major function of health education is empowerment.
- Health promotion is predominantly a proactive process. It is a process that is done *with* people not *at* people, either on an individual basis or within groups. Participation and partnership are key components of the process.
- Enabling people to take control is not as simple as saying, for example, 'it's up to you to make a choice', or 'it's your responsibility'. The latter approach directs total responsibility toward the client and assumes understanding, accurate interpretation and an ability to make inferences about the information received.
- Health promotion is said to work best for all members of society if it seeks to tackle the socioeconomic and environmental arena in which individuals live their everyday lives.
- Social capital is concerned with health promotion at this level and involves the forging of partnerships which encourage, enhance and value social relationships.

References

Bhatti T 1997 The effectiveness of alliances of partnerships for health promotion. A global review of progress and potential consideration of the relationship to building social capital for health. Conference working paper, 4th international conference on health promotion. WHO, Geneva

Biriotti M 1997 Tomorrow's world. Healthline 45:18–19

Bradshaw J 1972 The concept of social need. New Society 19:640–643

Bright J 1997 Health promotion in clinical practice. Baillière Tindall, London

Caplan R, Holland R 1990 Rethinking health education theory. Health Education Journal 49(1):10–12

Curie C, Todd J 1992 Health behaviours of Scottish school children: Report 1: National and regional patterns. Health Education Board for Scotland/Research Unit in Health and Behavioural Change, Edinburgh University Press, Edinburgh

Department of Health (DOH) 1992 Offering voluntary named HIV antibody testing to women receiving antenatal care. DOH, London

Dimond B 1994 The legal aspects of midwifery. Books for Midwives Press, Cheshire

Dines A, Cribb A 1993 Health promotion; concepts and practice. Blackwell Science, Oxford

Downie R S, Tannahill C, Tannahill A 1996 Health promotion models and values. Oxford University Press, New York

Ewles L, Simnett I 1999 Promoting health, a practical guide, 4th edn. Baillière Tindall, Edinburgh

Flay B, McFall S, Bioton D, Cook T, Warnecke J 1993 Health behaviour changes through television. Journal of Health and Social Behaviour 34:322–335

Gillies P, Spray J 1997 Addressing health inequalities: the practical potential of social capital. Health Education Authority, London

Harrison E F 1987 The managerial decision making process. Houghton Mifflin, Boston MA

Langer E J 1983 The psychology of control. Sage, Beverley Hills, CA

Leap N 1991 Helping you to make your own decisions: antenatal and postnatal groups in Deptford, SE London (VHS video)

Lewis L 1986 The concept of control; a typology and health related variables. Health Education 3(1)

Naidoo J, Wills J 1998 Practising health promotion. Dilemmas and challenges. Baillière Tindall, London

Rawson D 1992 The growth of health promotion theory and its rational reconstruction. In: Bunton R, Macdonald G (eds) Health promotion disciplines and diversity. Routledge, London, pp 202–224

Tannahill A 1985 What is health promotion? Health Education Journal 44:167–168

Taylor R 1979 Medicine out of control: the anatomy of a malignant technology. Sun Books, Melbourne

Tones K 1981 Health education: prevention or subversion? Royal Society of Health Journal 3:114–117

Tones K 1991 Health promotion, empowerment and the psychology of control. Journal of Health Education 29(1):17–21

Tones K 1992 Empowerment and the promotion of health. Journal of the Institute of Health Education 30(4):29–30

Unlinked Anonymous Surveys Steering Group 1997 Prevalence of HIV in England and Wales – 1996. Annual report of the unlinked anonymous HIV prevalence monitoring programme; England and Wales. Department of Health, Public Laboratory Services, Institute of Child Health, London

Vuori H 1980 The medical model and the objectives of health education. International Journal of Health Education 23:1–8

Wilkinson R G 1996 Unhealthy societies. The afflictions of inequality. Routledge, London

World Health Organization (WHO) 1984 Health promotion: a discussion document on concepts and principles. WHO, Geneva

World Health Organization (WHO) 1986 Ottawa charter for health promotion. Journal of Health Promotion 1:1–4

Yeo M 1993 Toward an ethic of empowerment for health promotion. Health Promotion International 8(3):225–235

Recommended reading

Gillies P 1998 Effectiveness of alliances and partnership for health promotion. Health Promotion International 13(2):99–117

This paper offers the reader a broad view of promoting health and reducing health inequalities. Partnership initiatives to promote health and tackle the broader determinants of health and well being in populations is the discussion point of this paper. Social capital is cited as a framework for promoting health and reducing inequalities.

Kelly M 1996 Code of ethics for health promotion. The Social Affairs Unit, St Edmundsbury Press

Seedhouse D 1997 Health promotion: philosophy, prejudice and practice. John Wiley, New York

This critical exploration of health promotion presents many challenges to those working in the field of health and health promotion and any other agency claiming to promote health.

3 Understanding the nature of behavioural change – foundations for practice

Key themes

- Behavioural change considered within the individual's social, cultural and economic position
- Attitudes and attitudinal change
- Beliefs and their influence on behavioural change
- Behavioural change during pregnancy
- Theories of behavioural change

Overview

This chapter explores the factors which influence behavioural change from a social psychology perspective. Theoretical models which seek to predict and explain changes in health behaviour will be highlighted and discussed in terms of efficacy. An appreciation of the complex process involved in behavioural change is useful when planning health promotion initiatives. The reader should be able to reflect on previous health promotion strategies used when facilitating behavioural change and consider the efficacy of the approach, based on the theoretical models discussed.

The discussion of the concept of health and its different meanings presents challenges for the varied scope of health promotion work. Integral to this is the notion of behavioural change, which is defined as encouraging change towards the adoption of a healthy lifestyle (Stott, Kinnersley & Rollnick 1994). Health care professionals may benefit from regular education updates on how to facilitate this process. It is a fallacy to believe that the provision of information alone influences a change in behaviour. This idea not only assumes that the individual has the freedom to choose, but also assumes that people are able to think rationally at all times and make rational decisions based on information received. The Research Unit in Health and Behavioural Change (1989) suggests that action is a consequence of emotion, habit and impulse and not purely cognition. Psychological theories and models have sought to understand and predict how and why people make lifestyle changes. Behavioural change is often treated as a process that is separate from social influence, with the onus of responsibility placed on the individual to make lifestyle changes. If the change is not made, or not maintained, the burden of guilt is left with the individual. Strategies used by the individual to deal with feelings of guilt and failure may include an increase in or resumption of the behaviour the health promoter sought to change, for example an increase in the number of cigarettes smoked. Health professionals should therefore consider behavioural change within the context of individuals' cultural norms and the socio-economic circumstance in which they conduct their everyday lives.

Attitudes

A person's attitude influences, to a large extent, how health promotion initiatives are received and the nature of behavioural change which follows. Due to the problems identified in determining a definition of attitude, the process of change is problematic. It is clear however, that attitudes are not fixed, nor determined at birth, and are therefore susceptible to change. An attitude is formed through experience and is not necessarily consciously learned. Attitudes which are supported and approved by others become stronger and therefore more difficult to influence and change. If the attitude is inconsistent with the individual's cultural group then group influence may cause a change in attitude. This change may be short or long lasting and is largely determined by how much the individual values the cultural group.

Attitudes may or may not determine behaviour. This is an important reality for behavioural change strategies and the adoption of healthy lifestyle choices. The promotion of breast feeding is a useful example; research evidence suggests that this is the best food available for the newborn baby. As such, the enthusiasm by which this information is promoted may encourage the adoption of the behaviour but not a change in attitude. As a consequence the behaviour is short term, with the client's intention being to suit the request of the midwife. Individuals tend to respond or act in accordance with how they believe others want them to, which does not always reflect their true attitude. An alternative approach to increasing the breast-feeding rates involves client-centred health education, which provides the opportunity to explore health beliefs. In this situation the attitude is more likely to be congruent with behaviour. In the first example the cognitive depth of the message (i.e. the midwife's enthusiasm for the benefits of breast feeding) was superficial and socioeconomic and cultural influences were not considered. The second example is a demonstration of cognitive depth, and is considered to be relatively stable (Downie, Tannahill & Tannahill 1996). Wilson & Colquhoun (1998) suggest that attitudes are likely to determine behaviour. They state that when women meet midwives their feeding intentions are clearly established and professional procedures are not always able to offer effective intervention.

Attitudinal change

Heider's theories of cognitive consistency (Heider 1944) present an argument based on people organising their beliefs and attitudes between tension states and tension free states. People generally strive to be comfortable with their own attitudes, beliefs and perceptions, thus enabling a tension free state. If cognitions are challenged the individual's state becomes one of tension and as such the person is motivated to adjust to a non-tension state. Heider suggests that only after becoming aware of the tension can the individual strive to adjust to a tension free state and classifies this as the balance theory (Heider 1958). The adjustment may result in: a change in cognition, a blocking out or rejection of the matter causing the tension or redefining a part of, or the whole, cognition. Either way a tension free state is assumed. The balance theory does not predict which outcome may occur, however; this was clarified by Festinger's (1957) cognitive dissonance theory. Cognitive dissonance is said to exist when a person holds two cognitions that contradict each other. This theory enables the prediction of how people will behave if forced to do something that is contrary to their belief. The theory also has the potential to influence a change in attitude and/or behaviour. Cognitive dissonance is an antagonistic state which motivates people toward an agreeable state of consonance, through either attitudinal or behavioural change. This dissonance also helps to explain the facet of communication where people communicate to receive information which supports cognitive consonance. This type of selective dialogue may be used to bury painful memories and/or used to reinforce beliefs about a situation which was unavoidable. An element of self-blame or blame of others is utilised to resolve dissonance. Consider the case study in Box 3.1.

Socially mediated experiences involve learning from the consequences of other people's behaviour, which can also cause attitudinal change, or an attempt to reinforce and strengthen existing attitudes. Consider the case study in Box 3.2.

Discussion question

- Think of areas of your work where attitudes and beliefs of the professional and the client influence health outcome.
  In light of Heider's theories of cognitive consistency, how can you use these principles to improve your work?

Beliefs

Belief has been defined as follows: 'What one has been told, or what one

Box 3.1 **Case study: Tara**

Tara's baby had died after she admitted herself to the labour ward complaining of reduced fetal movements. Although there was a detectable heart beat on admission to the labour ward, there were obvious signs of fetal distress. A caesarean section was organised and within 8 minutes a live baby was delivered, with low Apgar scores. After advanced resuscitation the baby was certified as dead.

A year later Tara had still not come to terms with her baby's death. First, she blamed herself because she had smoked throughout her pregnancy; she blamed her partner for not helping her to stop smoking; she eventually focused the blame on the midwives and the doctors for not saving her baby.

At a local support group Tara sought information from other mothers who had had similar experiences. The focal point of her communication was the length of time it took from the decision to carry out a caesarean section to the time the baby was born. The dialogue she had with the bereavement counsellor constantly sought for issues surrounding response times to caesarean sections. She avoided talking about her own guilt feelings and her anger toward her partner.

Tara sought to maintain consonance in order to avoid mental pain.

Box 3.2 **Case study: Sarah**

Sarah is 15 weeks' pregnant and smokes 25 cigarettes a day. She smoked during her two previous pregnancies, which resulted in the delivery of low birthweight babies. Sarah described them as being cute and healthy. She believes that the same will happen this time and having a smaller baby is easier because labour is easier. Although she acknowledges the detrimental effects of smoking toward herself and her baby, she feels that the baby is somewhat protected, she seeks to rationalise her behaviour based on her own experience, her mother's very similar experience and her sister who smoked throughout all five pregnancies and delivered average weight babies.

Consider the following approaches to health education in terms of efficacy;

- The midwife provides Sarah with overwhelming evidence about the effects of cigarette smoke on the fetus, which is inconsistent with her current beliefs. The midwife seeks to clarify Sarah's ideas about smoking, encouraging her to identify damage limitation strategies. She also discusses Sarah's thoughts about low birthweight babies and informs Sarah of real life examples of smoking and adverse pregnancy outcome.
- The midwife gives Sarah leaflets on stopping smoking made easy and informs Sarah of the new hospital policy which forbids any smoking inside the hospital or within its grounds. She reminds Sarah that from admission to discharge she will be unable to have a cigarette.

discovers, that has no basis in current experience, or any such form of knowledge that exerts some control over thoughts, actions, perceptions and motives is referred to as a belief' (Claxton 1988). A belief is therefore based on cultural information received from birth and influence from significant others, usually without any challenge. Beliefs which are conceived from experience and continue throughout adult life are less receptive to change. Claxton (1988) refers to four commonly held beliefs which have a direct influence on behaviour: I must be competent, I must be consistent, I must be in control, I must be comfortable. The principles of this idea are commonly cited as obstacles to behavioural change and the fear of failure. Schwarzer & Schwarzer (1996) suggest that, whilst believing that a particular change in behaviour is likely to increase health, it is important to encourage self-efficacy. The behavioural change approach to health promotion should therefore include the process of empowerment as an integral strategy to achieving the overall aim. This serves to reduce reliance on medical control and influence.

Behavioural change during pregnancy

Behaviours which are injurious to health are often enjoyable to the client and used as a coping strategy to relieve life stresses. Benefits of the behaviour are therefore often perceived as outweighing the risks. For example, smoking and drinking alcohol are enjoyable to the client, considered to be least of all addictive and form part of a social culture. Behaviour cannot be changed without consideration of the context in which the behaviour occurs. Pregnancy is viewed as a stressful life event for some women; therefore removal of the coping behaviour they have learned to rely on, for example smoking, may be detrimental to their emotional and mental well being. Others view pregnancy as a new beginning and, as such, are more receptive to behaviour change. As discussed earlier, self-efficacy is an essential part of the health promotion process. Communication skills which encourage exploration of thoughts and feelings will highlight contextual barriers and enable the health professional to utilise the relevant and appropriate intervention strategies. Feelings of despondency and poor productivity may be experienced by the midwife if behavioural change is not achieved. It is important to remember that the process of health promotion work is equally as important as the outcome. The potential to raise awareness and empower people to make choices should not be underestimated, and may encourage individuals to place behavioural change higher on their personal life agenda.

Changes in patterns of behaviour are influenced by a number of factors. There may be no logical progression to behavioural change, since the influence that drives the behaviour may be deeply rooted in culture, religion, or purely a mix of emotion, habit, impulse, addiction, social deprivation, poverty and/or a need for social acceptance. There continues to be discussion about why some people adopt healthy lifestyles and others do not, despite the same health promotion strategy and similar socioeconomic circumstances of recipients. One theory of health-related behavioural change offered a plausible explanation. This theory, proposed by the Research Unit in Health and Behavioural Change (1989), purports that everyday life activities fall into predictable patterns of everyday life for any given individual and form part of routine. The process of learning the behaviour encourages cognition whereby the behaviour is a salient part of the individual's consciousness. With repetition, however, it forms part of routine, becomes overlearned and is carried out with little cognition, coming to the forefront of consciousness in a superficial way. Although once voluntary, the behaviour then becomes fixed and inflexible due to overlearning. Once the behaviour is incorporated into routine habitual behaviour, the higher levels of consciousness are freed to deal with more salient features of everyday life (Luria, Simernitskaya & Tubylevich 1970). Schutz (1970) suggests that only very superficial levels of self are involved in superficial acts like eating and drinking, and refers to them as 'quasi-automatic' chores. It is thus postulated that acts like smoking and alcoholic drinking form part of this group of chores when regular indulgence takes place. They are therefore not salient to the individual engaging in the activity. This lack of salience is suggested to have implications for the perceptual processes of the individual concerned, as follows. Perception is the result of a summation which takes place between incoming information and internal processes. Issues which reach conscious attention are selected based on their interest, value and relevance. The selectivity of our perception therefore has an influence on how health messages are received: they may be vaguely received therefore but are not selected as subjects for conscious attention, unless they have become salient for that individual because of some other reason.

It should therefore be possible to create a set of minimum conditions under which changes of health-related behaviour are likely to take place. A prerequisite for change is that the subject must become salient to the individual in a way which encourages exploration of meaning in the context of everyday life. For instance, the context in which the change is occurring should be appropriate. Also, the climate of support should be flexible and adaptable to reduce the person's perceived barriers to the change process.

Theories of behavioural change

Various models have been developed over the years to help predict and understand behavioural change. At the very least they encourage critical thought and provide a theoretical framework in which to start to work. Environmental health issues are an influencing factor on the determinants of health, as are economic and political constraints, and as such these factors should be considered when using the following models.

Health locus of control

Rotter's theory of 'locus of control' is commonly used for exploring how people's beliefs about health and illness affect what they do (Rotter 1966). This assumes that how people explain what happens to them is based on their learning experiences. It assumes, for instance, that individuals who were rewarded for good behaviour and punished for bad behaviour during their formative years come as adults to view their successes as just rewards for hard work rendered. They feel that they are responsible for and control their own behaviour and are viewed as having an 'internal locus of control'. In contrast, however, those people who were rewarded or punished unmethodically during their formative years view life circumstances as being inevitable and as a consequence of good or bad luck. They are described as having an 'external locus of control'. Rotter's work was adapted by Wallston, Wallston & De Vellis (1978) who included a third category of people who attribute their health to 'powerful others'. This refers to the belief that the actions of doctors and other health professionals determine health outcomes through instructions, recommendations and medication they provide. The theory was thus labelled a multidimensional health locus of control scale. This model has been used to recognise and accept an individual's existing belief about health outcomes and to provide information according to their belief, in order to promote health behaviour. By noting a patient's responses to multidimensional health locus of control items, a health professional may be able to identify the pattern of orientation as being related more strongly to belief in internal control or control by powerful others. Using this information as a guideline, the professional could strive to present advice about screening behaviours, in line with the patient's existing multidimensional health locus of control orientations.

This model has been heavily criticised and has failed on many occasions to explain how people's beliefs about health and illness affect what they do (Wallston & Wallston 1981). It allows little room for flexibility and as such promotes a rigid regimen for health strategies based on three categories of assessment. It also suggests that the experiences of chilhood are never influenced by later experiences, which may thus change the locus of control. Norman et al (1998) carried out research utilising the classification of Wallston & Wallston's (1981) locus of control typology. Eleven thousand six hundred and thirty-two people completed a questionnaire measuring health locus of control, health value and a number of health behaviours.

A health behaviour index was formed after combining measures of smoking, alcohol consumption, exercise and diet. The results were positively associated with internal health locus of control scores and negatively associated with scores on the influence of powerful others. The researchers suggest that the value placed on health moderates the relationship between health locus of control and health behaviour. They conclude that the health locus of control, by itself, is a weak predictor of health behaviour and suggest the need to consider other expectancy beliefs when attempting to predict health behaviour. The possibility that values other than health values also determine the performance or non-performance of health behaviour deserves further attention. For instance, Kristiansen (1987) advocates the use of relative health measures as predictors of healthy behaviour, and purports that the health behaviour of young people is more likely to be predicted by their own personal values than by a standard health index value which involves long term health gain.

The following two examples are health behaviour theories which are commonly described as 'continuum theories'. They are concerned with identifying variables which influence action, which are then combined in a predictive equation. Each theory has a single prediction equation and as such the way behaviours combine to influence action is expected to be the same for everyone (Weinstein & Rothman 1998). Behaviour does not necessarily progress in the same sequence and follow the same process. Although commonalities may be apparent between groups of people, individuality is lost.

Reflection point

- Reflect on aspects of your work where your intention has been, through health promotion, to change a client's behaviour. Think about the behavioural change theories read so far and discuss with your colleagues how the principles can be applied to achieve your aim.

The health belief model

The health belief model was originally developed in 1966 by Rosentock and was later modified by Becker in 1974. It was developed specifically to explain and predict how individuals would behave in relation to their health. Participation in matters relating to preventative health behaviour is predicted on the basis of the individual's perception of: the person's susceptibility to a given disorder, the seriousness or severity of the disorder, the benefits of taking action, the barriers to action and the cues to taking action (Becker 1974). An individual's beliefs about whether they are likely to contract an illness and the degree to which they perceive an illness as being severe is sometimes referred to as a perceived threat and is the basis by which behaviour is influenced. Modifying factors may include sociocultural factors, age and gender. The model suggests that people will think about the advantages and disadvantages of engaging in health behaviour, even if the existing behaviour is not changed and relies on a particular cue for action to be taken. This could be in the form of a health scare, advice from others or a major life event. Unfortunately, some people believe that they will not become ill, as they perceive certain illnesses to happen only to others. Pregnancy, for example, is often seen as a cue for smoking cessation (Dunkley 1997). The model has also been criticised for the equal weighting given to different factors; for example all the barriers to taking action, regardless of their nature and cultural significance, are equally weighted (Naidoo & Wills 1998).

Theory of reasoned action

Ajzen & Fishbein's (1980) theory of reasoned action is based on the assumption that most human behaviour is under voluntary control and is therefore largely guided by intention. The theory considers the individual's attitude towards a behaviour as well as the influence of the social environment as important predictors of behavioural intention. The social norms of groups can therefore influence intention, and can be used positively during antenatal group education to influence the adoption of, for example, breast feeding. The midwife's attitude toward breast feeding may also be viewed as a powerful influence toward adopting the behaviour, as previously discussed. Intention can therefore be driven by the attitude of significant others. Beliefs and intentions are not always predictive of behaviour. The theory is criticised predominantly for this reason as it does not account for behaviour that occurs outside of the realms of prediction and intention, which is considered its major drawback (Research Unit in Health and Behavioural Change 1989). Ajzen & Fishbein (1980) acknowledge that the intention of the individual does not always cause the intended behaviour. The behaviour may be different to the intention and is largely influenced by the strength of the belief by which the intention is determined. Transient beliefs are more indicative of dissonance between intention and behaviour. Attitudes of significant others and subjective norms of groups may influence intention, which may be short term. In summary, this theory acknowledges social factors, peer pressure, media influence, the socioeconomic and the political context in which individual intention toward behaviour is guided.

Stage theory of health behaviour

Stage theories attempt to stop unhealthy behaviour. They are used to identify the dominant stage and stages of changes in health behaviour and focus resources on those issues that would progress people to the next stage. The theories assume that change in health behaviour proceeds through a series of stages and, as such, treatments and the sequence of treatments need to be matched to the individual needs of people (Weinstein & Rothmam 1998). To assess whether behavioural change does progress through stages, Weinstein & Rothmam (1998) suggest that consideration of four defining properties of a stage theory of health behaviour is necessary:

- **A classification system to define the stages.** Stage of health behaviour are divided into categories, with very little differences between the characteristics of the behaviour of different people within the stage and diverse differences between people in different stages.
- **An ordering of the stages.** This is concerned with specifying the sequence of the stage. People are viewed as individuals within the stage and may therefore progress through subsequent stages. This may happen very quickly because they have the essential components, or people may stay in the stage for a considerable length of time if the essential components for change are lacking.
- **Common barriers to change facing people in the same stage.** This feature of a stage theory of health behaviour is concerned with people in the same stage sharing commonalities with others, and as such interventions which are applied to one person may be useful to others in the same stage.
- **Different barriers to change facing people in different stages.** This feature acknowledges that some barriers are more important at certain stages than others.

The theorists conclude that defining the stages and specifying their sequence are the initial steps that seek to demonstrate that health behaviours progress through stages. The ultimate test is concerned with discovering the barriers between the stages and showing the benefits of using different interventions as people move through the stages. A stage model is useful in helping to identify intervention only if it is possible to ameliorate or influence the factors which influence the progression of behaviour from one stage to another.

Reflection point

- Reflect on aspects of your work where your intention has been, through health promotion, to change a client's behaviour. Think once again about the behavioural change theories read so far and discuss with your colleagues how the principles can be applied to achieve your aim.

The behavioural change model

The model of behavioural change is the most widely used stage model in health psychology. It was originally developed by Prochaska & DiClemente (1992) to examine smoking cessation behaviour. It is now widely used for a wide range of behaviours, including smoking, alcohol and drug abuse, dietary changes and exercise. The model is useful in identifying stages of behavioural change. It offers the possibility of creating programmes and treatments that meet the specific needs of each identified stage of behaviour. It also recognises that for some people change may involve cycling through these stages more than once. (See Ch. 6 for this model related to practice.)

Modification of addictive behaviours involves progression through five stages as follows.

- **Precontemplation**. This is the stage at which there is no intention to change behaviour in the foreseeable future. Many individuals in this stage are unaware or underaware of their problem. It is suggested that they can see the solution but cannot see the problem (Prochaska, DiClemente & Norcross 1993).
- **Contemplation**. This is the stage in which people are aware that a problem exists and are seriously thinking about overcoming it, but have not made a commitment to take action. People can be stuck in the contemplative stage for a great deal of time.
- **Preparation**. This is a stage which combines intentional and behavioural criteria. Individuals in this stage are intending to take action in the next month and have unsuccessfully taken action in the past year.
- **Action**. This is the stage in which individuals modify their behaviour, experiences or environment in order to overcome their problems. Action involves the most overt behavioural change and requires considerable commitment of time and energy.
- **Maintenance**. This is the stage in which people work to prevent relapse and consolidate the gains attained during action. Being able to remain free of the addictive behaviour and being able to consistently engage in a new compatible behaviour for more than 6 months are criteria to classify an individual as a maintainer (Prochaska, DiClemente & Norcross 1993). Such an arbitrary figure as criteria for maintenance deems anything less than this period as failure or relapse. Establishing a new compatible healthy behaviour can be difficult and only when that behaviour becomes habitual can maintenance be prolonged.

Self-change of addictive behaviours involves external influence and individual commitment. Professionals frequently design excellent action-orientated treatment and self-help programmes, but are then disappointed when only a small percentage of people register, or when large numbers drop out of the programme after registering. It is important to remember that overambitious demands will inevitably be frustrating.

Using this model may reduce the potential for coercion, which is sometimes used to promote behavioural change. Attempts to coerce or encourage changes in behaviour may be counterproductive and increase resistance or resentment (Stott, Kinnersley & Rollnick 1994). Readiness to change must be taken into account. This varies both within and between individuals. Evidence is emerging that the practitioner's approach should be more sensitively matched to the client's readiness to change. For example, while an action-oriented smoking programme may help those who are ready for change, it does not help those who are unsure about it (Prochaska & DiClemente 1992). Those who are unsure need not advice but the opportunity to weigh up the advantages and disadvantages of changing their behaviour. Trying to assess the readiness to change also has the merit of focusing on the person rather than the message.

Discussion question

- The behavioural change model is commonly used for smoking cessation work. How can this model be used in other areas of your work to facilitate the process of behavioural change?

Critics of the model have expressed concern that it is not clear what proportion of people who successfully deal with an addiction progress in an orderly way through the posited stages of change. In a longitudinal study Prochaska & DiClemente (1992) followed 180 smokers, who were initially in the contemplation stage. Of the 180 self-changers, only nine demonstrated a strictly linear pattern of behaviour change over a 2-year period. The most frequent response was to remain stuck in contemplation for the entire 2 years. Other common patterns involved action (cessation), followed by relapse. Recycling through the stages or regression back to an earlier stage of change would then follow (Prochaska & DiClemente 1992). The researchers suggest that it is possible for individuals to successfully leap over stages, for example, from precontemplation to maintenance, but this was not evident in the study. Individuals who leap to action without adequate contemplation or preparation were at high risk of relapse.

Although the model does not contribute to knowledge about the nature, aetiology and development of addictive behaviour, it allows for assessment and evaluation. It enables practitioner autonomy and ensures greater parity between the agendas of the practitioner and the client. This will help to minimise the emergence of resistance and improve the effectiveness of the intervention (Stott, Kinnersley & Rollnick 1994)

Summary

- Understanding the nature and context of human behaviour is the starting point for the modification of individual habits.
- Health professionals should consider behavioural change within the context of individuals' cultural norms and the socioeconomic circumstance in which they conduct their everyday lives.
- A person's attitude influences to a large extent how health promotion initiatives are received and the nature of behavioural change which follows.
- Behaviours which are injurious to health are often enjoyable to the client and used as coping strategies to relieve life stresses.
- The potential to raise awareness and empower people to make choices should not be underestimated, and may encourage individuals to place behavioural change higher on their personal life agenda.
- Various models have been developed over the years to help predict and understand behavioural change. At the very least they encourage critical thought and provide a theoretical framework from which to start work.
- Models which seek to understand and predict behavioural change may be used as a guidance or framework but ultimately an individualised approach to enhancing the change process will ensure efficacy.

- Health promotion and health education strategies can only truly influence the adoption of healthy lifestyles when people's lives become less strained and free from socioeconomic disadvantage, which at its worst encourages the reliance on behaviours perceived by them to be stress relieving but are in fact health destroying.
- Deprivation and disadvantage are clearly political issues. Although it can be argued that health will not be achieved nor illness minimised unless the inequalities which exist between nations and within nations and social groups are tackled successfully, at local level health professionals cannot do everything but what is done must be done effectively.

References

Ajzen I, Fishbein M 1980 Understanding attitudes and predicting social behaviour. Prentice Hall, Englewood Cliffs NJ

Becker M H 1974 The health belief model and personal health behaviour. Thorofare, New Jersey

Claxton G 1988 Live and learn, an introduction to the psychology of growth and change in every day life. Open University Press, Milton Keynes, pp 47–49

Downie R S, Tannahill C, Tannahill A 1996 Health promotion models and values. Oxford University Press, New York

Dunkley J 1997 Training midwives to help pregnant women stop smoking. Nursing Times 93(5):64–66

Festinger L 1957 A theory of cognitive dissonance. University Press, Stanford CA, pp 60–64

Heider F 1944 Social perception phenomenal causality. Psychological Review 51:358–374

Heider F 1958 The psychology of interpersonal relations. Wiley, New York, pp 92–101

Kristiansen C M 1987 Social learning theory and preventive health behaviour. Some neglected variables. Social Behaviour 2:73–86

Luria A, Simernitskaya E, Tubylevich B 1970 The structure of psychological processes in relation to cerebral organisation. Neurological Psychology 8:217–231

Naidoo J, Wills J 1998 Practising health promotion. Dilemmas and challenges. Baillière Tindall, London

Norman P, Bennett R, Smith C, Murphy S 1998 Health locus of control and health behaviour. Journal of Health Psychology 3(2):171–178

Prochaska J, DiClemente C 1992 Stages of change in the modification of problem behaviours. In: Hersen M, Eisler R E M (eds) Progress in behaviour modification. Sycamore Press, pp 184–214

Prochaska J, DiClemente C, Norcross C 1993 In search of how people change: applications to addictive behaviours. Addictions Nursing Network 5(1):2–16

Research Unit in Health and Behavioural Change 1989 Changing the public health. John Wiley, Chichester

Rosentock I 1966 why people use health services. Millbank Memorial Fund Quarterly 44:94–121

Rotter J B 1966 Generalised expectancies for internal versus external control reinforcement. Psychological Monographs 80(1)

Schutz A 1970 Reflections on the problem of relevance. Yale University Press, New Haven CT

Schwarzer R, Schwarzer C 1996 A critical survey of coping instruments. In: Zeidner M, Endler N S (eds) Handbook of coping: theory research, applications. John Wiley, New York, pp 107–132

Stott N C, Kinnersley P, Rollnick S 1994 The limits to health promotion. British Medical Journal 309:971–972

Tones K 1992 The theory of health promotion, implications for nursing. Paper presented at the International Nursing Conference, King's College, London, September

Wallston K A, Wallston B S 1981 Health locus of control scales. In: Lefcourt H M (ed) Research with the locus of control construct, 1, assessment methods. Academic Press, New York

Wallston K A, Wallston B S, De Vellis R 1978 Development of the multidimensional health locus of control scales. Health Education Monographs 6:161–170

Weinstein D, Rothman A 1998 Stage theories of health behaviour: conceptual and methodological issues. Health Psychology 17(3):290–299

Wilson D, Colquhoun A 1998 Influences in the decision to breast feed: a study of pregnant women and their feeding intentions. Nutrition and Food Sciences 4 (July/August):185–192

Recommended reading

Weinstein D, Rothman A 1998 Stage theories of health behaviour: conceptual and methodological issues. Health Psychology 17(3):290–299
A comprehensive guide to understanding health behaviour from a theoretical perspective.

Communication, counselling and the midwife

4

Overview

Communication and counselling skills remain the single most important aspect of health promotion work. The effectiveness and efficiency of health promotion strategies are therefore influenced by appropriate and skilled communication.

This chapter aims to highlight basic communication skills, barriers to communication and the nature and value of counselling and the counselling relationship. Counselling takes years of study and requires practice and participation. An in-depth examination of communication and counselling skills is beyond the scope of this chapter but can be explored in greater detail by utilising the suggested reading list. Throughout the following pages, health professionals are encouraged to reflect on their experiences of communicating health promotion and consider how professional and client communication barriers can be reduced when health promotion becomes the focal point for discussion.

Communication – progress and change

During the last 20 years there have been published reports highlighting problems of poor communication. Failure of the communication process is a frequently complained about aspect of maternity care. Complaints can be used to improve services and highlight the need for training in communication skills (DOH 1994a). The Maternity Services Advisory Committee (1982) recognised the need for improved communication as a means of making the maternity services approachable and accessible. To enhance good communication skills during the antenatal, intrapartum and postnatal period, communication guidelines and a communication checklist was developed. The committee felt that this would enable clients to ask questions freely and have them answered appropriately and sensitively. A decade later the Department of Health published the Patients' charter (DOH 1991), which briefly addressed the right of the patient to receive a clear explanation in order to make informed choices about proposed health care. Due to limited relevance to pregnant women within the charter, the National Childbirth Trust (NCT) (unpublished study, 1992), suggested that there should be a separate charter to address the specific needs of pregnant women. The Patient's charter maternity services (DOH 1994b) was therefore published; it clearly details the needs and requirements of maternity service users with regards to effective communication. The Winterton report (DOH 1992) focused on the experiences of pregnant women and highlighted poignant areas of poor communication. The report stated that pregnant women often experience an 'unwillingness on the part of health professionals to treat them as equal partners in making decisions' (DOH 1992 para 73). Recommendations thus followed detailing strategies to improve communication skills. Finally the Changing childbirth report (DOH 1993), adopted as government policy in 1994, allocates a whole document to a survey of good communication practice in the maternity services. It identifies areas of strengths and areas for improvement and includes effective communication as an integral part of the report's indicators of success.

What is good communication?

In its narrowest sense communication involves the passing on or transfer of information. This can be done either verbally or through the expression of non-verbal behaviour. Non-verbal behaviour is open to individual subjective scrutiny, more so than verbal interpretation. How people communicate is primarily based on their previous life experiences, culture, attitudes, values and belief systems. Argyle (1992) states that cultural differences of non-verbal behaviour are a major source of misunderstanding and aggravation. Good communication is essential for successful health promotion, but it is difficult to define. It involves the provision of clear, unambiguous exchange. The receiver of the message should receive the identical message that the sender intends. A distortion of the theme may be the result of incongruent non-verbal behaviour, so it is important that facial expression and speech are congruent. Once a message has been sent, be it verbally or non-verbally, it cannot be retracted, as it has already been received. Ellis, Gates & Kenworthy (1995) suggest that every action or non-action communicates something. A model showing the complexities involved in communication is presented in Figure 4.1. This model acknowledges the uniqueness of individual perception, in line with social and cultural differences, and views communication from the intrapsychic world, which is indicative of thoughts and feelings, and the interpersonal world, which is indicative of interaction with other people. The thoughts and feelings of the sender are encoded into verbal and/or non-verbal behaviour; the receiver then decodes and interprets the message before sending a response, again of a verbal and/or non-verbal nature. Regardless of the intent of the message, the decoding process, which is dependent on how the message is perceived, will determine the response.

Reflection points

- Reflect on your experiences of poor communication. In which could communication have been improved?

- Identify times when as a result of poor communication your efficiency at work was reduced. How did this make you feel?

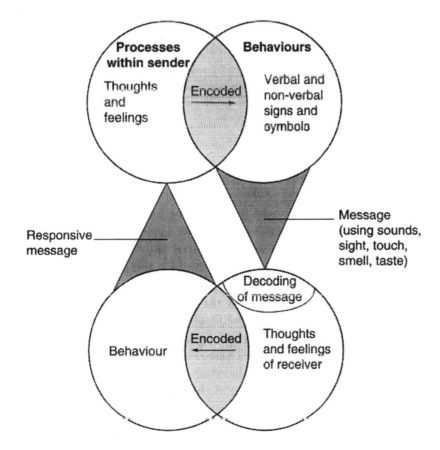

Figure 4.1
A model of communication (from Ellis, Gates & Kenworthy 1995, with permission)

One-way and two-way communication

The conveyor belt analogy of the busy antenatal clinic is indicative of one-way communication and cannot meet the aims and objectives of antenatal care. In the past the focus of communication between the midwife and the woman was one sided in order to impart traditional health education (Royal College of Obstetricians and Gynaecologists & Royal College of Midwives 1995). Conversely, the maternity booking interview, although criticised for its overzealous aim of providing women with large amounts of information, assumes an interactive two-way communication process. Ellis, Gates & Kenworthy (1995) highlight the fact that many who express agreement with two-way communication in theory do not practise it. Two-way communication provides the opportunity for feedback, which has the potential for clarifying how the message was received. Two-way communication enables the midwife to develop a therapeutic relationship with the woman. This is described as communication which is supportive, healing and interactive in nature (Pearson 1991). Interpersonal skills involved in this process include empathy and trust and, if communicated, form the basis of a helping relationship (Bradley & Edinberg 1990). This process forms an integral part of midwifery practice and reflects the current philosophy of midwifery care. Identifying needs encourages the development of working strategies. Providing information, giving advice, teaching and taking action are examples of helping which require good communication skills. A skilled helper, however, utilises conditions of empathy, genuiness, respect and confidentiality (Egan 1994), the qualities of which are developed through effective communication skills.

Barriers to communication

Discussing certain health promotion issues may encourage communication barriers, owing to the nature of the subject raised. The most popular health promotion approach to be used by midwives includes health education, empowerment and behavioural change. For instance, consider a session discussing smoking cessation with a woman and her partner who each smokes 30 cigarettes per day. Both enjoy smoking and have no desire to give up. Midwives may find it difficult to explore smoking cessation and damage limitation issues, possibly because of the fear of creating communication barriers and destroying the midwife–client relationship. Equally the woman and her partner may feel challenged about a behaviour they enjoy and see no potential for harm. This may result in limited discussion which is unable to raise awareness or ameliorate behaviour. An unpublished study carried out by Dunkley in 1997 found that midwives who were involved in smoking cessation counselling of pregnant women stated their concerns about destroying their relationship with the woman as a reason for not discussing and exploring the subject in detail. In addition, midwives who were smokers themselves very often felt hypocritical about counselling women on smoking cessation.

When recording a woman's obstetric history midwives should ask 'open' questions, which allow clients to express fears, worries and anxieties. Establishing open dialogue early in the booking or antenatal visit can help reduce communication barriers which are often perceived when subjects warranting behavioural change are addressed. An inability to provide this basic prerequisite to effective health promotion may render delicate issues, which require a relationship of honesty and trust, to be explored in an environment which is closed and non-receptive. An understanding of the role of health promotion in today's maternity services should encourage communication that supports self-empowerment, client autonomy and the provision of accurate, appropriate research-based information. Women and their families will then be given the opportunity to explore and discuss health lifestyle options and ultimately make informed choices.

Effective communication is largely determined by:

1. how professionals feel about themselves as individuals – their self-worth
2. how the professional views the client/how the client views the professional
3. the professional's knowledge base about the subject
4. the language used.

1. Self-worth

The ability to communicate is partly determined by how individuals feel about themselves. Those with low self-esteem are said to be more critical of themselves and underestimate their abilities, which is subsequently reflected in the communication process (Ewles & Simnett 1999). Increasing self-awareness in these areas may result in improved communication. Being self-aware is considered to be the first step to effective communication (Burnard 1994). Attempting to become more self-aware in isolation of others may lead to a subjective personal assessment and thus be open to personal bias. The process of self-awareness must involve feedback from others as well as the ability to be introspective – that is, to step outside and observe oneself objectively (Burnard 1994). Stress may also adversely affect the ability to communicate effectively and may be expressed in a manner which debilitates the communication process.

It is merely an assumption that all health professionals are able to communicate effectively and appropriately. How often have you heard the following?

- 'Of course we communicate well; we provide current, referenced, research-based information for women to read.' (Providing written information does not equal two-way communication. An overreliance on leaflets and handouts represents misuse. Such information utilised appropriately reinforces two-way communication, but it is not intended to replace it. The RCOG & RCM (1995 p. 34) state that 'It is not uncommon for a pregnant woman to leave a hospital antenatal clinic with a sheaf of information of miscellaneous literature – but with no idea of the significance of the check up she has just had.' A study carried out by Jacoby in 1988 revealed that reading was the most commonly cited way of receiving information from the midwife in the antenatal period.)
- 'We are always seeking to improve our communication channels by, for example, reading the woman's birth plan.' (Reading a birth plan only is not effective communication. Discussion about the content, reassuring and supporting ideas, clarifying and reaching a suitable compromise are all integral to the aim of the birth plan.)
- 'We do not have a problem with communication, there was just a misunderstanding.' (Misunderstandings involve communication.)
- 'You can tell by the woman's body language when you try to discuss smoking that she is getting defensive.' (Consideration also needs to given about the approach taken when discussing smoking cessation, see Ch. 6.)
- 'She's not really rude; once you get used to her you'll realise that she talks to everybody like that, and always has done, for as long as I have been here.' (Acceptance, collusion and dismissive comments do not improve obvious communication problems. These should be challenged.)
- 'How could they say that I was rude and uncaring when I did not say a single word; Sister Joyce can vouch for that!' (Non-verbal communication speaks volumes. It involves all forms of communication that do not include the spoken word. Gestures and body language are variable and are influenced by the environment and socioeconomic status (Sundeen et al 1998).)
- 'How could they say that they had to follow hospital policy; I always offer choice!' (Hospital policy is sometimes used in sentences when informing women about certain practices. Sometimes women are informed about the hospital policy and then asked to make a choice. Some women may find it difficult to request a type of care or approach that may differ from policy and as such may feel that they have no choice, because of the way the information was communicated.)

2. How the professional views the client/how the client views the professional

Midwifery has progressed toward reducing social barriers to communication but room for further progress is warranted. The Audit Commission report (1993) describes many areas where communication is deficient between users and providers of care. As social class is an outward sign of social status, it plays a significant role in the process of social relations (Jarvis 1984). Research which focused on communication in labour revealed that women of higher social classes asked for and received more information than women from lower social classes. The nature of the requests from women of lower social classes was unassuming and diffident in nature and therefore midwives made assumptions about what women would understand based on their social class (Kirkham 1989).

Stereotypes

Stereotypical ideas encourage communication to be influenced by subjective value judgements. Stereotypes are ideas, values and social rules that are perpetuated by society about individuals or groups. They are maintained and sustained by structures within society that are seen to hold power.

To challenge and change stereotypes to enable a realistic view of reality would involve an exploration of personal perceptions and those of others. A clear knowledge of self and self-awareness is a necessary pre-requisite to challenging personal stereotypical ideas. Messages can be distorted if midwives are not aware of their own prejudices, attitudes and belief systems (see Ch. 3). Accepting and understanding people's individual differences and adopting a non-judgemental approach to communication, regardless of the decisions made by the client, enhances the communication process. The client, however, may view the midwife as being critical or judgemental if communication is one way. Equally, previous bad experiences of midwives and/or childbirth can negatively influence the communication process. Clashes of personality may be apparent, in which case intermediary support from colleagues may be necessary. Developing a good relationship with the client which involves two-way communication is very often maintained by mutual admiration and respect between the client and the midwife. Acknowledging strengths, praising progress and overcoming difficulties are important factors when maintaining the relationship.

Incongruence

Incongruence involves verbalising a message whilst portraying a behaviour that is incongruent with the verbal message. The message received is therefore distorted and confused. An example of a situation when an incongruent message may be evident is the typical busy period on an ante/postnatal ward where service needs are greater than care providers. The portrayal of 'busy' behaviour is often inevitable. During such times, despite the friendly inviting tone of voice from the midwife, the communication received by the client is non-verbal busy behaviour. Questions, fears and anxieties are either not aired, aired only when a problem arises or saved for the student midwife or student nurse, who are perceived as less busy. A barrier to communication has thus been created. Sundeen et al (1998) suggest that non-verbal communication that accompanies speech involves a complexed coordination of pausing, looking, head nodding, smiles and gazes. Clients may also view non-verbal cues, including frowning, avoiding eye contact and an obsessive relationship with case notes, as an exhibition of non-caring and abstract behaviour; this seeks to inhibit a trusting relationship between themselves and the midwife.

Consider the case study in Box 4.1. In this situation, Jade displayed incongruent behaviour and did not communicate with Lisa honestly and effectively. Very often, 'don't worry' is seen as a platitude offered to women and is a negative command which has very little meaning. When observing communication between the midwife and the woman in labour, Kirkham (1989) identified words like 'don't worry' as an attempt to allay the woman's fears; it was seen as a tool for quietening and for making the midwife feel that she had resolved the situation. The midwife's ability to listen is an essential part of the communication process. Careful listening reveals aspects other than the spoken word including the tone of voice. Careful observation may reveal body language which demonstrates disagreement and anxiety. Listening and observation will enable the midwife to become more focused and in tune with the woman's communication

---

Box 4.1 **Case study: Jade**

Jade is a midwife who was in Lisa's home carrying out her antenatal booking visit. She had allocated herself ample time to conduct the booking visit at ease. Lisa, who was expecting her second baby, had only consulted her general practitioner about the pregnancy at 33 weeks' gestation. Her first baby unfortunately was in foster care. The booking was going extremely well with Lisa asking lots of questions and discussing her fears and anxieties. Jade was supportive and knowledgeable and responded well to Lisa's needs. Jade suggested that she listen to the baby's heart beat prior to abdominal palpation. Unfortunately Jade could not find the heart beat with the pinnards stethoscope, her facial expression was one of worry, her rush to get the hand-held Doppler caused Lisa concern and she began to panic. So, although Jade reassured her verbally and told her not to worry, her facial expression was incongruent as she searched for her hand-held Doppler, turning to frustration and then panic. She told Lisa that the Doppler must be in her car and reassured her once again that everything was fine. Lisa was convinced that something was desperately wrong as Jade's body language was panicked and distressed. Whilst Jade had gone to the car Lisa called her partner in panic and requested that he come home. Unfortunately Jade had parked two streets away and took time to return. Once Jade returned with the hand-held Doppler she hurriedly listened to the fetal heart. The fetal heart pounded out loud and clear at 140 beats per minute.

pathway and thus communicate more effectively. Busy schedules and workloads inevitably influence the quality of the communication but awareness of how this is perceived should encourage reflection and subsequent improvement. A need for further training in communication and counselling adapted to meet the current needs of maternity services, together with regular update sessions, begs serious consideration. This is supported by a study which aimed to identify the educational needs of midwives and found that counselling and communication skills featured high on the agenda of midwives and supervisors of midwives, who expressed a need for training and update (Pope et al 1998).

3. The professional's knowledge base

Discussing a health issue with little knowledge of the subject is loaded with problems. Not only can it limit the depth and nature of the discussion, but a poor knowledge base reduces the client's choices, owing to the limited amount of information received. Failure to communicate effectively and appropriately may result in the client's consent being totally invalid, leaving the midwife's actions classified as trespassing (Dimond 1994). A limited knowledge base may encourage professionals to choose not to hear certain questions or rush conversation along rather than acknowledging what has been asked. Knowledge instils confidence and enables the midwife not only to provide competent advice and information but to instil confidence and trust in the client.

Lack of current evidenced-based knowledge is also likely to cause conflicting advice to be given to the client. Conflicting advice is likely to lead to confusion and influence the client's receptiveness to the health message. Losing public confidence by providing conflicting advice has the potential to encourage mistrust and disapproval and cause the client to view further health messages with scepticism.

Families and friends may contradict information given by the midwife, which also adds to confusion.

4. Language

The use of professional terminology to lay members of the public mystifies ideas about pregnancy and childbirth and reinforces professional dominance. Equally, interpreting and understanding colloquial language can cause problems and should therefore be avoided. Dialects and subdialects used within particular languages may confuse the meaning of words. Jargon must be avoided; this principle is well known and fundamental to effective communication, yet at times jargon is still used. Sometimes it is used unconsciously; at other times it may be used to mystify, impress or dominate people. Using language in this way as been described by Ellis, Gates & Kenworthy (1995) as an example of sending multiple messages where the hidden message is of prime importance over and above its surface meaning. All communication must be directed at a level which the client and her family can understand.

Improving communication

Attention to the following areas may help to improve communication skills. (Empathy and genuineness, commonly referred to as core conditions, are addressed later within the context of a counselling relationship.)

Increasing self-awareness

Gradually exploring aspects of self and recognising differences and similarities in the context of the internal world of thoughts, ideas and feelings and the external world may help increase self-awareness (see Fig. 4.1). Improving awareness of personal attitudes, beliefs, values and behaviour is likely to result in a more constructive use of self. Burnard (1994) argues that, at its best, developing self-awareness can help to have a better understanding of others.

Improving listening skills

Listening is a fundamental aspect of effective communication. It is generally described as a passive process of receiving information. Burnard (1994), however, contends that listening is an active state characterised by being alive, within the spectrum of the individual's communication. This involves both mental and physical commitment. Listening involves maintaining eye contact, open body posture, maintaining close proximity but respecting spatial needs and nodding in appropriate places. This not only demonstrates interest in what the person is communicating, but also acknowledges receipt of the information. Awareness of different cultural behaviours during communication will enrich the process further and reduce the chances of portraying behaviour which is deemed disrespectful. Effective listening can encourage clients to continue to communicate freely and feel that their opinions/contributions are valid and worthwhile. To improve listening skills Van Dersal (1974) suggests that three questions should be borne in mind during listening: what does the speaker mean? how does the speaker know? and what is being left out?

• **What does the speaker mean?** The midwife should be aware of the different meanings attached to words by different cultural groups, for example: 'I have never had an abortion. I have had one baby that was abnormal, so they started the labour when I was 5 months, and took it away'.

• **How does the speaker know?** This question alerts the midwife to listen for the reasons behind the information being given to enable an understanding of who or what circumstance has influenced the client.

- **What is being left out?** This question will alert the midwife to information that has been vaguely given, partly given or assumed that the midwife already knows.

Paraphrasing is a useful technique to clarify meaning. This involves repeating what the client has said, but rephrased, and helps the midwife derive more from the listening process. Clients will then have an opportunity to clarify misunderstandings or express precisely what they intended to say initially. It is important to note that clients may still remain vague, or omit to disclose information clearly, during initial meetings with the midwife until such time that they consider the therapeutic alliance within the relationship to be good.

Mirroring may also be used to enhance listening skills. It involves reflecting back what the client has said, word for word. This not only reassures clients that they are being listened to but also enables midwives to remain cognitively sharp and alert when it is necessary to listen for long periods of time.

Reflection

Reflection can enhance communication skills by encouraging evaluation and thought about the communication interaction. Van Manen (1991) and Boud, Keogh & Walker (1994) describe several types of reflection including 'active' reflection, which is thinking during the event, and 'mindfulness' reflection, which is described as being involved thoughtfully in a situation where active consciousness takes place but is open to true reflection only after the event. Midwives may be able to reflect in action by processing what is happening during an interaction without waiting until afterwards. The benefits to be gained from reflection in action include positive thoughts and feelings that serve to support the interaction when it is viewed to be going well and an increase in options and adjustment in strategy, which can help to ensure that the outcome of communication is successful. However, reflection in action offers an opportunity to address the situation if things are not going to plan only if there is accurate processing of the information.

Learning from feedback

Dickson, Hargie & Morrow (1989) describe feedback in both the intrinsic and the extrinsic sense. Intrinsic feedback involves individuals observing and listening to the responses of the person or people to whom they are communicating. Non-verbal and verbal behaviour is received and internalised (see Fig. 4.1). This type of feedback, however, is prone to subjective interpretation and as such is not a valid form of feedback when used alone. Extrinsic feedback is the receipt of information from others based on the interaction; it may be either verbal or written. It is suggested that both types of feedback are fundamental elements to improving communication and enable a critical look at self, a different perspective other than personal assumptions, reinforcement of positive aspects of the communication and information for further reflection.

Improving communication through audit

Auditing of the communication process enables the recognition of good practice, highlights areas for improvement, enables the recognition of training need, and assesses compliance to The patient's charter (DOH 1994b) and the progress toward performance indicators and indicators of success. Overall auditing of the communication process ensures good practice, maintains high standards and ultimately ensures the provision of a quality service.

The audit committee at the Royal College of Obstetricians and Gynaecologists and the Royal College of Midwives (RCOG & RCM 1995) developed standards for communication between health professionals and pregnant women for audit purposes. The document provides a practical guide to audit, giving ideas for evaluating the content of communication as well as the process. The areas suggested for audit address social, cultural and ethnic differences. The overall aim of the document is to improve standards of communication. The audit committee also endorses the use of complaints about standards in communication to improve services.

Reflection points

- How do you propose that communication and counselling skills could be improved in your area of work?

- How do you audit communication in your place of work?

- How are the results of the audit used?

Counselling

There are many instances when the relationship between the midwife and the woman is one where the midwife uses counselling skills but does not engage in a counselling relationship. Midwives are often involved in counselling prior to and after an HIV test, or crisis-orientated counselling, for example after an intrauterine death, or stillbirth. It is often the midwife who is involved in the debriefment process after childbirth, which will inevitably involve utilising counselling skills (see Ch. 9). Therapeutic value for the woman and her family will also be an integral part of this process. Indeed any situation which is perceived as traumatic to the woman may result in the midwife offering some kind of therapeutic support. A large proportion of midwives' work involves empowering women to make choices; an integral part of this process is the utilisation of skills which encourage a client-centred non-directive approach. It is for this reason that an appreciation of counselling theory may broaden midwives' scope and understanding of the helping role they find themselves in. It is useful to recognise the difference between utilising counselling skills in a helping relationship and engaging in a counselling relationship. Role identification reduces the chance of role confusion.

A counselling relationship is described as a formal counselling contract and the counsellor has no other role in relation to the client (McLeod 1993). Lack of clarity between the two roles may cause difficulty not only for the client but for the midwife, particularly when the midwife chooses to leave the counselling relationship and continue with other work. One midwife can have a multiplicity of roles including that of health promoter, manager, supervisor, teacher and counsellor. It is essential that the nature of each encounter is clearly understood by both parties if serious role confusion is to be avoided. An agreed definition of the nature of counselling would also be beneficial and the rules that apply during this time.

Drapela & Victor (1990) argue that it is not helpful to draw professional lines of demarcation under which midwives cannot engage in a counselling relationship with clients if they feel that they have the expertise to do so; however, exceeding professional capabilities is not advisable (United Kingdom Central Council (UKCC) 1998). It is important, however, to recognise when to refer clients for specialist counselling. This may include the following situations:

- when the needs of the client exceed the expertise of the midwife
- when the client can be helped more effectively by established specialist agencies
- when the client is suicidal
- when the client is severely depressed.

If there is a need to refer a client for counselling, it is important to reassure them that referral does not signify closure of the midwife–client relationship. The client should be motivated toward accepting the help which is deemed to exceed the midwife's professional capabilities. Direction and help during the referral process should be facilitated by the midwife and agreed to by the client.

The aim of using counselling skills is to facilitate the client through a process which enables personal growth and development, raises awareness, encourages a deeper look at self and others and facilitates the ability to take charge and cope. This may involve: exploring choices, making decisions and therapeutic healing. The overall outcomes of a counselling relationship are summarised by Egan (1994 p. 7) as follows.

1. Effective helping results in something valued being in place that was not in place before the helping session(s).
2. Unreasonable fears will disappear or diminish to manageable levels.
3. Self-confidence will replace self-doubt.
4. Addiction will be conquered.
5. An operation will be faced with a degree of equanimity.
6. A better job will be found.

Reflection points

- Consider the above description of a counselling relationship (McLeod 1993) in light of your current working role.
- Reflect on aspects of your work which involve counselling.
- Reflect on the number of occasions you have entered into a counselling relationship.
- How can the counselling role of the midwife be clarified?

7. A new life will be breathed into a marriage.
8. Self-respect will be restored.

The midwife may be able to identify with the outcomes two, three, four and eight, which may be evident, for example, after exploring hopes and fears related to pregnancy and labour and discussing strategies which empower individuals to have a sense of control and self-efficacy. Similarly individuals who smoke may be successfully counselled toward smoking cessation.

Non-directional client-centred counselling

The client-centred approach to counselling utilises a range of skills that may be modified by midwives to facilitate a therapeutic helping relationship with clients.

The Rogerian approach to counselling involves counsellors restricting themselves to the role of facilitator and consciously refraining from any activity which may direct the client. If any insight is then achieved it has come from the client and not from the counsellor (Rogers 1974). This approach is referred to as 'non-directional client centred'. It works to its full potential when relevant and helpful recognition and resolution are what clients discover for themselves and relate to the context of their world. It is suggested that any intervention by the therapist to manipulate the client, however good their intention, contradicts the client-centred theory (Merry 1990). Owen (1990) challenges this assertion and states that it is difficult to be in a close relationship whereby one person fails to influence the other. The client will therefore be influenced by the counsellor despite the counsellor's non-directive approach. 'Behavioural counsellors' question the notion of a non-directional client-centred approach and suggest that it assumes that clients have the necessary skills to deal with non-direction (Owen 1990). Midwives as skilled helpers may have difficulty adopting a totally non-directional approach. Some clients specifically ask for direction, sometimes during moments of stress, tension and pain when they view support as guidance and request this from the midwife. The non-directive approach may, however, be utilised during circumstances where the situation and environment warrant the utilisation of counselling skills (see Fig. 4.2). Some clients are aware of the choices that are available to themselves as consumers and are totally capable of self-direction.

Rogers (1974) sees conditions such as empathy, congruence and unconditional positive regard as important conditions necessary for successful counselling and therapeutic change. He describes therapeutic change as a 'process of greater openness to experience' where the client has increasing awareness of denied experience and movement from perceiving the world in generalisations. He states that the client and counsellor must be in contact and congruent in the relationship. The client must perceive the counsellor's unconditional regard and empathy because if these are not perceived they do not exist as far as the client is concerned and there will be no move toward autonomy by the client and subsequent change. This theory was tested by many researchers (Gallagher & Hargie 1992, Gurman 1978, Klassen & Turgeon 1981); their results have shown that each of the relationship variables were in isolation insignificant in bringing about therapeutic client change. Also wide variations were found in the clients' and counsellors' views on 'empathy', 'congruence' and 'unconditional positive regard', which were also found to be difficult to measure.

Rogers conceptualised the process of counselling as a series of stages to increase clients' involvement in their inner world (McLeod 1993). The seven stages of increasing client involvement in the inner world involve: stage one – communication, stage two – expression, stage three – describing personal reactions to external events, stage four – descriptions of feelings and personal experience, stage five – present feelings, stage six – flow of feelings, and stage seven – a series of felt senses connecting different parts of an issue. Research has shown that clients who begin therapy at level one of this model are less likely to be able to benefit from the process. The whole process is said to be facilitated by empathy, congruence and unconditional positive regard of the counsellor. This process can take some time within a counselling relationship and is very rarely achieved on the initial interaction.

The qualities of the counsellor

Rogers (1974) views the core conditions of: empathy, genuineness, respect and confidentiality as pre-requisites for meaningful help to take place. Although they are not totally exclusive to the success of a helping relationship, they form essential components. Withers & Wantz (1993) carried out a study which investigated the influence of belief systems on subjects' perceptions of empathy, warmth and genuineness expressed by the counsellor. The data indicate that individuals' perception of a therapist whom they have only observed, are significantly influenced by their belief systems. It is suggested that the most appropriate interventions will be utilised by developing a better understanding of the counselling style and the client's belief system. Owen (1990) states that the counsellor and the client come from two different worlds and as such interpersonal difficulties may be apparent. Cultural differences are also acknowledged and within the context of the counselling relationship it is suggested that ethnocentricity may also be apparent – that is, holding on to culturally bound views and believing them to be true, and another person's untrue. Acceptance, flexibility, recognition of the client's culture, being aware of internal and external contexts and stepping out of one's own internal context will enhance the counselling relationship, by causing the counsellor to adapt to different clients as opposed to simply his or her natural self (as supported by the client-centred approach). The serious implications involved in cultural stereotyping should, however, be avoided. It is suggested that the differences within a culture are as great or greater than the differences between cultures (Schott & Henley 1996). Within a culture the ideas about social and economic influences still apply, and therefore absolute categories and generalisations in order to understand cultural groups are counterproductive.

It is suggested that one of the important aspects of a counselling relationship is the internal and external contexts of the client and the counsellor, which are assumptions of the Rogerian approach. In order to create appropriate care the counsellor needs to have a good appreciation of the client's understanding (i.e. the client's culture). To gain this understanding counsellors must step out of their own internal context, which may involve previous experiences of the client, the counsellor's state of mind and beliefs, etc. This would enable counsellors to have a flexible objective approach.

An in-depth study into the range of skills used in counselling is beyond the scope of this chapter, but the main skills can be summarised in Figure 4.2. This illustration of counselling skills also identifies reflection as the central theme for effective helping. To maintain and/or attain effective counselling skills, reflection on each skill can lead to an effective and appropriate integration of them.

The skilled helper

Egan (1994) proposes a model called the 'skilled helper', which is described as a systematic approach to helping. This model presents a practical approach to managing problems which warrant counselling skills. The model presents three stages of the helping process: present, future and getting there. Each stage is subdivided into sections which require progression from one stage to the next in a linear sequence. The model encompasses several aspects of the Rogerian approach to counselling, but does not explicitly demonstrate that individuals may return to the different stages, owing to its linear approach. The sections for progression in skilled helping include: exploration and clarification, identification of blind spots, facilitating focus, setting out possibilities, goal setting, commitment, strategies and plans. Each section is compartmentalised, 'which suggests an inflexible process to helping and does not acknowledge the unpredictable nature of

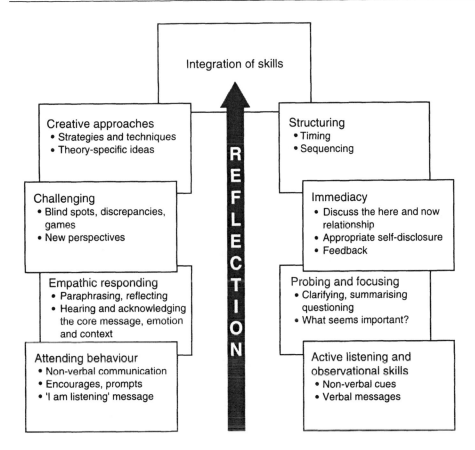

Figure 4.2
**Counselling skills
(from Ellis, Gates &
Kenworthy 1995, with
permission)**

human emotion. The model may, however, be useful as a framework for raising awareness of the multiplicities involved in a helping relationship and present a behavioural approach for those who are new to the concept of skilled helping.

Empathy

Empathy can be defined as 'the ability to sense the client's world as if it were your own, but without losing the as if quality' (Kalisch 1971 p. 203). This definition highlights the need to remain objective whilst understanding the world from the other person's perspective. The helper then remains in a position to help. The ability to empathise is not complete unless the health professional is able to communicate that understanding actively to the client. The empathy cycle as proposed by Barrett-Lennard (1962) suggests that there is an interconnectedness of the core conditions and suggests that the counsellor is not making use of separate skills, but instead is offering the client a whole personal relationship between them.

Empathy can contribute to the overall helping process in a variety of ways. The counsellors without prejudgements or assumptions allow themselves to be open to perceive the world as their clients perceive it (Egan 1994, Greengross 1986). Egan acknowledges, however, that the skill of the helper and the state of the client can have a bearing on the effectiveness of the process.

Confusion between empathy and sympathy is often apparent and should be avoided. Consider the case study in Box 4.2. Midwife two attempts to be caring and empathetic but is in fact caring and sympathetic. The response fails to acknowledge Olun's pain and the fact that she referred to her baby as a special baby. Although midwives view all babies as special, each client has their own personal feelings. Midwife two speaks from a position of paternalism and closure by reassuring Olun that 'we' will sort things out. This can also be viewed as taking control away from a situation where Olun feels that she has no control. Midwife one offers an empathetic and skilled response by acknowl-

---

Box 4.2 **Case study: Olun**

Olun arrived on the labour ward frantic with worry. She was expecting her first baby and was 34 weeks' pregnant. Olun had not felt the baby move for the last 24 hours. She approached the labour ward desk where one midwife was writing in case notes (midwife one) and a second midwife was opening the drug cupboard (midwife two). The conversation progressed as follows:

Olun: 'My name is Olun, I have not felt my baby move for some time.'

Midwife two: 'Don't worry I'll be with you in a minute; are we expecting you?'

Olun did not answer; the midwife finished checking the drugs and settled Olun into a room. Unfortunately the midwife could detect no fetal heart beat; this was confirmed by ultrasound scan. Olun broke down and became hysterical. Midwife one entered the room to provide moral support. Midwife one asked Olun if there was anybody she could telephone. Olun could not reply as she was so upset. After approximately 3 minutes of Olun crying hysterically the conversation continued as follows:

Midwife two: 'I'm so sorry I'll just get you some tissues and a cup of tea.'
   Olun: 'No, no, don't go. I cannot believe that my baby is dead. This baby is a very special baby; I cannot cope with all this. Why me?'
   Midwife two: 'I really don't know, these things sometimes just happen. Don't worry, we'll get this sorted out for you.' (Midwife two leaves the room.)
   Midwife one: 'This baby is such a special baby for you; it is difficult to believe that this has happened. Coping can be difficult but we will be here to support you.'

edging her feelings and not attempting to move things on toward closure.

It is assumed that health professionals have the ability to empathise. Ellis, Gates & Kenworthy (1995) challenge this assumption and argue that if, during childhood, a child does not abandon its egocentric view of the world experienced during normal child development and move toward acknowledging the different subjective experiences of others, then the ability to empathise with others in later life will be difficult (Ellis, Gates & Kenworthy 1995).

Genuineness

Genuineness is sometimes referred to as congruence and is described by Rogers (1974) as counsellors recognising their own feelings and ensuring that the inner experience matches with the outer expression. Genuineness is concerned with integrity and not a plastic performance or routine role. It is said to help the client receive clear messages from the counsellor and gain confidence from the counsellor's honesty. Egan (1994) suggests that the key principles related to genuineness include: being consistent, open, spontaneous but tactful, able to receive criticism without becoming defensive and not overemphasising the helping role. A client who perceives that the relationship between the helper and herself is genuine is able to progress toward developing trust and therapeutic change.

Respect

Egan's (1994) ideas of respect comprise valuing people because they are human, and suggest that no other criterion is necessary. Respect therefore remains constant, with no room for prejudice or discrimination. This ideal viewpoint provides a standard for helpers to recognise differences between themselves and their clients but remain non-judgemental. The process of socialisation often encourages individuals to make judgements about others, making the non-judgemental approach difficult. Exploration of self and awareness of personal attitudes and beliefs which may form value judgements can therefore help to preclude the entry of judgemental behaviour during a counselling interaction.

Confidentiality

Although confidentiality is the most fundamental aspect of the helping relationship, midwives have a professional responsibility to breach this if clients pose a risk to themselves. The client should be made aware of this prior to the start of the helping relationship.

Summary

- Good communication is essential for successful health promotion, but it is difficult to define. It involves the provision of clear, unambiguous exchange.
- Two-way communication enables the midwife to develop a therapeutic relationship with the woman. This is described as communication which is supportive, healing and interactive in nature.
- Stereotypical ideas encourage communication to be influenced by subjective value judgements. Stereotypes are ideas, values and social rules that are perpetuated by society about individuals or groups. Stereotypes are maintained and sustained by structures within society that are seen to hold power.
- Audit of the communication process enables the recognition of good practice, highlights areas for improvement, enables the recognition of training need and assesses compliance to The patient's charter and the progress toward performance indicators and indicators of success.
- Trained counsellors take many years to become expert and sometimes take equally as long to work through the intricate and complicated psychological traumas their clients face.
- Midwives may learn from counselling theories and techniques to improve and develop the counselling skills used within their work. Counselling skills underpinned by the appropriate theory can help the client and the midwife to progress toward therapeutic growth.
- The Rogerian approach to counselling is a client-centred non-directive approach which facilitates therapeutic growth by the counsellor expressing empathy, congruence and unconditional positive regard. It is concerned with clients knowing their own direction and answers and thus is client centred. Critics of the Rogerian approach to counselling encourage lateral thinking to those learning the approach; as Owen (1990) suggests this could enrich the whole process.
- It is useful to recognise the difference between utilising counselling skills in a helping relationship and engaging in a counselling relationship. Lack of clarity about the difference between the two roles may cause confusion and difficulty. Encouraging self-disclosure and being unable to cope with the results is unjust; therefore recognition of the need for specialist referral should form part of the midwife's helping criteria.
- A skilled helper utilises conditions of: empathy, genuineness, respect and confidentiality; these qualities are developed through effective communication skills.

References

Argyle M 1992 The social psychology of everyday life. Routledge, London

Audit Commission 1993 What seems to be the matter: communication between hospitals and patients. HMSO, London

Barrett-Lennard G T 1962 Dimensions of therapists' response as causal factors in therapeutic change. Psychological Monographs 76 (43, no. 562)

Boud D, Keogh R, Walker D 1994 Reflection: turning experience into learning. Kogan Page, London

Bradley J C, Edinberg M A 1990 Communication in the nursing context. Appleton & Lange, Connecticut

Burnard P 1994 Counselling skills for health professionals, 2nd edn. Chapman & Hall, London

Department of Health (DOH) 1991 The patient's charter. DOH, London

Department of Health (DOH) 1992 Maternity services government response to the second report from the Health Committee, session 1991–1992

Department of Health (DOH) 1993 Changing childbirth: the report of the Expert Maternity Group, parts 1 and II. DOH, London

Department of Health (DOH) 1994a Being heard: the report of a review committee on NHS complaints procedures. DOH, London

Department of Health (DOH) 1994b The patients' charter maternity services. DOH, London

Dickson D, Hargie O, Morrow N C 1989 Communication skills training for health professionals: an instructor's handbook. Chapman & Hall, London

Dimond B 1994 The legal aspects of midwifery. Books for Midwives Press, Cheshire, England

Drapela, Victor J 1990 The value of theories for counselling practitioners. International Journal for the Advancement of Counselling 13(1):19–26

Egan G 1994 The skilled helper. Brooks/Cole, Pacific Grove, CA

Ellis R, Gates R, Kenworthy N 1995 Interpersonal communication in nursing theory and practice. Churchill Livingstone, New York

Ewles L, Simnett I 1999 Promoting health, a practical guide, 4th edn. Baillière Tindall, Edinburgh

Gallagher M, Hargie O 1992 The relationship between counsellor interpersonal skills and the core conditions of client centred counselling. Counselling Psychology Quarterly 5(1):3–16

Greengross W 1986 Introducing counselling skills and techniques. Faber & Faber, London

Gurman A 1978 The patient's perception of the therapeutic relationship. In: Gurman P, Razin G (eds) Effective psychotherapy. Pergamon Press, Toronto, pp 17–20

Jacoby A 1988 Mothers' views about information and advice in pregnancy and childbirth: findings from a national study. Midwifery 4:103–110

Jarvis P 1984 Adult learning in the social context. Croom Helm, London

Kalisch B J 1971 An experiment in the development of empathy in nursing students. Nursing Research 20(3) (May–June):202–211

Kirkham M 1989 Midwives and information giving during labour. In: Robinson S, Thomson A M (eds) Midwives, research and childbirth, vol 1. Chapman & Hall, London, pp 117–138

Klassen D, Turgeon P 1981 The effect of Rogerian counselling conditions on locus of control. International Journal of Advanced Counselling 4:89–99

McLeod J 1993 An introduction to counselling. Open University Press, Buckingham

Maternity Services Advisory Committee 1982 Maternity care in action 1, antenatal care. Crown Copy, London

Merry M 1990 Client-centred therapy, some trends and some troubles. Counselling (February): 17–18

Owen I 1990 Re-emphasising a client centred approach. Counselling (August): 92–94

Pearson A 1991 Primary nursing. Chapman & Hall, London

Pope R, Cooney M, Graham L, Holliday M, Patel S 1998 Aspects of care 5: the continuing educational needs of midwives. British Journal of Midwifery 6(4):266–270

Rogers C 1974 On becoming a person. Constable, London

Royal College of Obstetricians and Gynaecologists (RCOG) and Royal College of Midwives (RCM) 1995 Report of the audit committee's working group on communication standards. RCOG and RCM, London

Schott J, Henley A 1996 Culture, religion and childbearing. A handbook for professionals. Butterworth-Heinemann, London

Sundeen S J, Stuart G W, Rankin A D, Cohen S A 1998 Nurse client interaction, implementing the nursing process, 6th edn. Mosby, London

United Kingdom Central Council (UKCC) for Nursing, Midwifery and Health Visiting 1998 Midwives rules and code of practice. UKCC, London

Van Dersal W 1974 How to be a good communicator and a better nurse. Nursing 4:58

Van Manen 1991 The tact of teaching the meaning of pedagogical thoughtfulness. University of New York Press, New York

Withers K, Wantz T 1993 The influence of belief systems on subjects' perceptions of empathy, warmth and genuineness. Psychotherapy 30(4):608–615

Recommended reading

Burnard P 1994 Counselling skills for health professionals, 2nd edn. Chapman & Hall, London

Department of Health 1993 Report of maternity services. Part 2: Survey of good communications practice in maternity services. HMSO, London
This survey provides evidence of the benefits of good communication in the maternity services.

Ivey A E, Ivey M B, Simek-Downing L 1987 Counselling and psychotherapy: integrating skills theory and practice. Prentice-Hall, Englewood Cliffs, NJ

Minardi H, Riley M 1997 Communication in health care. A skills based approach. Butterworth-Heinemann, Oxford
A review of counselling skills and techniques which offers a positive foundation for health work.

5 The value of preconception care

Overview

Preconception care is described as the passport to positive health during pregnancy. It is the all-encompassing care that women need prior to becoming pregnant. Preconception health is often affected by a combination of social, environmental, pathological and behavioural factors. The aim of care is to optimise the chances of conception, ensure the maintenance of a healthy pregnancy and promote a healthy outcome for the mother and baby. The midwife is the ideal health professional to provide preconception care. The obvious benefits with regards to continuity are unquestionable. Unfortunately, due to reduced resource commitment and financial allocation, the current provision of care is sparse. The provision of preconception care involves aspects of health promotion which include: health education, self-empowerment, health protection and behavioural change. It is a broad subject, encompassing complex issues, some of which are beyond the scope and remit of this chapter. The following text, however, presents an overview of the benefits of preconception care and the midwife's role in the provision of care. Prior knowledge of the following areas will enable the reader to understand the issues discussed in this chapter:

- the physiology of the menstrual cycle
- conception
- embryonic and fetal development
- aetiology of diabetes and phenylketonuria
- human immune deficiency virus, rubella and hepatitis.

The benefits of preconception care

Antenatal care may contribute to the reduction in maternal and neonatal mortality and morbidity rates. The provision of care provides women with a service that promotes physical and psychological well being and ensures the safe progression of pregnancy, towards the delivery of a healthy baby and well-adjusted mother. Risk assessment during the antenatal period has been successful in pre-empting potential complications which may adversely affect the health of the woman and fetus. The provision of antenatal care, however, often begins at a time when major organ development has taken place. Survey data demonstrate that one in four pregnancies ends in miscarriage and one in 36 babies is born with malformations (Atik 1994). The potential to influence factors which predispose to adverse pregnancy outcome is lost if antenatal care is the only service provided. During the prenatal period some couples continue to engage in social behaviours which have a tetrogenic effect on the developing fetus. Others may continue to be exposed to toxic drugs and chemicals and subjected to inadequate nutrition. Equally unplanned pregnancies may present similar problems. Pre-existing health problems have the potential to reduce the chances of pregnancy progressing to term and/or contribute to adverse pregnancy outcome. Care during the prenatal period is therefore extremely important and allows women and their partners the opportunity to optimise the conditions necessary for reproduction.

The increasing prevalence of unplanned pregnancies suggests that preconception care should be available and accessible to all women who have the potential of childbearing. Cefalo, Bowes & Moos (1995) suggest that this approach will enable appropriate time for identifying and treating potential risks, lifestyle modification and an opportunity to make informed decisions about future reproduction and the psychological and socioeconomical consequences of unplanned pregnancies. The links between unplanned pregnancy and poor birth outcome are unclear, but speculation linking risk factors associated with maternal socioeconomic circumstances, maternal and paternal behavioural risk factors and an inability to seek antenatal care are tenable (Hellerstedt et al 1998). Women who have conceived an unplanned pregnancy are therefore likely to have the same or greater risk factors than those who have planned

Reflection point

- Reflect on areas of your practice where you have provided health education. What was the aim of health education you provided and what was the potential to influence preconception health?

pregnancies. A study carried out by Hellerstedt et al (1998) concluded that women having unplanned pregnancies were less likely to alter behaviour associated with risk during pregnancy than women whose pregnancies were planned.

Preconception care benefits:

- all men and women of reproductive age
- healthy fertile couples who wish to give themselves and their children the best possible start
- men and women who have infertility problems
- women who have had single or recurrent spontaneous abortions
- women who have existing or previous high risk medical and/or obstetric history.

Availability and accessibility

Preconception care is not a new concept, but has slowly gained momentum over the last 25 years. The current provision of care is limited, it does not form part of routine practice and does not meet the needs of local communities. It is suggested that preconception care should be available and accessible to all who have the potential for childbearing and should form an integral part of primary care services (Cefalo, Bowes & Moos 1995, Marsack et al 1995, Wallace & Hurwitz 1998). As early as 1978, Queen Charlotte's Maternity Unit (London, England) set up a preconception care clinic to provide guidance and support to women and their partners planning a pregnancy. Eighty per cent of the women who attended the clinic over a 3 year period chose to seek counselling despite the lack of medical and poor obstetric risk factors. Attendance therefore may have been based on a desire to optimise the chances of conception, maintain a healthy pregnancy and deliver a healthy baby (Chamberlain 1980).

Preconception care and the midwife

Preconception care should be available to all women and their partners as an integral part of primary care services. The most suitable professionals to provide this service are midwives, although support from members of the primary health care team and specialist services would be invaluable. For many years midwives who are considered expert in the provision of maternity care have also provided some aspects of preconception care, outside of the domain of a preconception clinic. This at present is carried out in a variety of ways in as many different settings, with little uniformity and structure to planned programmes. This ad hoc approach renders audit difficult to achieve. Most midwives may be able to recall situations where the opportunity to act on information prior to the booking visit would have made a difference to the success of the pregnancy – for example, preconception advice in relation to rubella immunity or advice about increasing folate intake. Very often a back to front service is offered, whereby women may be informed of tetrogenic effects to the fetus after exposure, or when they are unable to act on the information until after the pregnancy. Women who are non-immune to rubella are advised to avoid exposure during pregnancy, whereas offering immunisation prenatally would be far more preferable. Risk assessment is an essential component of this service in which midwives are well versed.

The resources to fund preconception care are limited. The knowledge base of the midwife warrants extensive, current, research-based information to inform preconception practice. To provide an effective and appropriate service, updates or further training in specific areas of preconception health may also be necessary. An example of knowledge deficits has been highlighted by Mulliner (1995); a study assessing the nutritional knowledge of health professionals demonstrated that many of the midwives sampled (n = 77) were unsure when advising mothers about food scares and alternative diets, and acknowledged that they were able to offer only basic advice. The need for training above and beyond that received during basic training, with regular update workshops, will ensure that comprehensive relevant knowledge is utilised, instilling confidence in midwives to discuss dietary issues with clients. This is further emphasised in the 1992 King's Fund report, A positive approach to nutrition as treatment, and the 1994 DOH document, The health of the nation. A study which aimed to determine knowledge and attitudes of members of the primary care team and women of childbearing age toward preconception care found that both health professionals and women had good knowledge of preconception care. Unfortunately only 40% of all women surveyed considered preconception care to be essential, which suggested that the majority of women would not seek this type of care spontaneously (Wallace & Hurwitz 1998). This may be because of poor understanding of the aim of preconception care, or socioeconomic disadvantage, which presents a barrier to participation in care programmes. The majority of health professionals surveyed felt that the most appropriate way of delivering preconception care was opportunistically (that is, on any occasion when the woman has contact with the health professional). Most clients, however, felt that this approach would be inappropriate when consulting on a matter outside of the realms of women's health.

Reflection point

- Is it ethical to provide opportunistic preconception care in a primary health care setting?

Opportunities to provide preconception care

Health services which are widely available and easily accessible to provide preconception care services include:

- family-planning clinics, well women's clinics
- workplace occupational health and workplace health promotion units
- pregnancy-testing forums, with referral opportunities
- general practitioners' surgeries
- schools: the death rates of babies born to teenage mothers are more than 50% higher than the national average (Office for National Statistics 1997); it is suggested that 'good preconception care begins with adequate sex and parenthood education in schools – information learnt slowly over a period of time is more likely to have an impact than hasty health education given when a girl or woman finds she is pregnant' (Chapple 1991, p. 17).

Results of a preconception risk survey, administered after a negative pregnancy test visit, revealed that 94% of the study group reported at least one factor requiring further evaluation, counselling or intervention before pregnancy (Jack & Culpepper 1990). The researchers suggest that negative pregnancy test visits provide an opportunity for preconception risk assessment and counselling.

Preconception care – an example of a provisional service

Providing a provisional service may be the only option available for maternity units who do not offer preconception care. Audit and evaluation have the potential of providing evidence, which in turn could support the request for a complete service involving additional training for staff in subjects including nutrition, mineral metabolism, allergies and environmental toxins. Financial commitment toward laboratory services, medical support and specialist services would also be necessary. A multidisciplinary approach is essential, utilising the expertise of each professional discipline. A provisional service even in its infancy, could offer a highly flexible worthwhile programme. Many midwives at present offer a health education evening, or an early bird session for women in very early pregnancy, or for those thinking about becoming pregnant. This forum could be utilised as the starting point for a preconception care service (see Box 5.1).

Political support for an improved service

Although public health initiatives have had a huge impact on the population's health over the last century, a more specific approach and commitment from government should be presented to enable preconception care to be widely available and taken more seriously. The Health Committee of the House of Commons called for evidence on preconception

Box 5.1 **An example of a preconception class integrated into an existing health promotion/early antenatal education class**

Part 1, day 1
- Exploring fears and anxieties
- Noting individual client expectations
- Presenting the aim and objectives of preconception care
- Providing an overview of health promotion issues focusing on social and environmental hazards
- Exploring psychological and social readiness toward becoming pregnant
- Encouraging the completion of health screening forms to determine physical risk factors

Individual one to one work
- Discuss and explore completed health-screening forms and suggested routes and/or referrals for risk appropriate counselling and screening; this may include suggestions for some clients to be referred for genetic counselling

Part 2, day 1
- Screening workshop (this may involve the discussion of screening for infections, reasons why and risks to the pregnancy)
- Diet and exercise workshop (this may involve exploring the benefits of exercise for sedentary clients, discussing safety aspects of exercise during pregnancy for those who exercise regularly and dietary advice)
- Smoking and alcohol workshop (this may involve discussing the benefits of cessation and risk to conception, pregnancy and the fetus)
- Previous obstetric history workshop (this may involve discussing potential risks of obstetric problems and the implications for future pregnancies)
- Records of identified risks and suggested referral points for specific help and support

NB Midwives who have expertise in the above areas should be invited to lead the workshops; a dietician and physiotherapist would be valuable in providing expert advice or indeed leading a workshop.

services in the session 1990–1991. A report was produced recommending the need for the whole community to have access to preconception care and awareness raised about behavioural, pathological, environmental and social factors which affect the health of prospective parents and their subsequent offspring. The suggested channel for communication and counselling was a multi-agency approach including the HEA and primary health care professionals, with a large emphasis on family-planning clinics providing preconception advice. Schools were also thought to be a useful channel of communication, where children could be given information and guidance to make informed choices about issues including

Reflection point

- Primary care groups should provide direct means by which the primary care teams and other health and social care professionals lead the process of securing high quality care for local people. How can the midwife ensure through this process that preconception care becomes a priority area and forms part of the health improvement programme?

contraception, pregnancy and parenthood. Unfortunately the government response to the committee stated that devising specific programmes for preconception health would detract resources from the whole population without any corresponding benefits. The reality, however, is that uptake of services which are available and accessible to the community safeguards the health of future generations. The Health of the nation report (DOH 1992a) briefly mentions preconception care but does not discuss it in detail nor make any recommendations for the provision of the service. More recently, the government consultation paper, Our healthier nation (Secretary of State for Health 1998), makes no specific reference to the provision of preconception care, but suggests that, by targeting priority areas of ill health, other health benefits will be seen. Smoking cessation, regular physical activity and eating healthily are mentioned as part of the strategy to improve health and reduce inequalities in health. Indirectly, such proposals may influence the health of prospective parents, but the need for a specific commitment toward preconception care would be more beneficial.

Preconception care the Foresight way

The most renowned and successful preconception care programme is run by the Foresight Association, a registered charity for the promotion of preconception care. Foresight recommends that this type of care should start 6 months before conception.

Foresight and a medical committee have worked for 15 years to collate a researched, scientific preconception programme for health professionals to implement, in order to help clients achieve and maintain a healthy pregnancy. The programme consists of rigorous and thorough screening of the woman and her partner, including: allergy, malabsorption and/or intestinal infestation, sweat tests and hair mineral analysis, followed by an individually planned health correction programme including Foresight vitamins and minerals. Research by the University of Surrey (England) on the Foresight programme presented interesting and promising results. The outcomes of 367 couples who had enrolled on a Foresight preconception care programme during 1990–1992 formed the population for the study. Toward completion of the study 89% of the couples had given birth. The average gestational age was 38.5 weeks and the average birth weight was 7 lb $4\frac{1}{2}$ oz (3.3 kg) for boys and 7 lb $2\frac{1}{2}$ oz (3.25 kg) for girls. There were no miscarriages, perinatal deaths or congenital abnormalities. Eighty-nine per cent of the study population had a range of reproductive, general health and age problems, some of whom smoked and drank alcohol and had previous obstetric histories, including miscarriage, infertility and previous small for dates offspring. Starting the programme involved changing behaviour considered to be 'risky', for example smoking and drinking alcohol. The results of the study, although promising, failed to demonstrate cause and effect relationships between variables; its external validity therefore is questioned. Also, the chances of socioeconomically disadvantaged groups engaging on the Foresight preconception care programme are limited as the financial cost may render the programme inaccessible.

Discussion question

- Reflect on the antenatal risk assessment sheets currently used in clinical practice. How may risk factors identified benefit from preconception care?

Risk assessment

Preconception care counselling involves identifying potential risk factors and discussing strategies to decrease or remove the risk. Risk assessment may include screening for the following factors.

Behavioural factors

Smoking

Smoking, alcohol and narcotics have a detrimental effect on the ova and sperm during the period leading up to conception and teratogenic effects on the fetus if a pregnancy is conceived. Evidence suggests that cigarette smoking may affect male fertility by altering spermatogenesis, sperm mobility and sperm morphology. Associations have been found between smoking and infertility, menstrual disorders, spontaneous abortions, low birth weight, infant mortality and infant morbidity (Cefalo & Moos 1988). Research has indicated that mothers who smoke during pregnancy increase the risk of their subsequent female infants giving birth to a child who is not of optimal health (Hawkes 1994). Not only are health interventions appropriate but their timing is very important. One in four pregnancies ends in miscarriage, usually in the first trimester (Atik 1994). Preconception care may not prevent this from happening, but may demonstrate a significant impact on its prevalence. In addition effective intervention programmes can have a significant impact on smoking behaviour and encourage the maintenance of a smoke free lifestyle (Dunkley 1997). (Ch. 6 offers a more detailed approach to smoking cessation.)

Alcohol

There is no internationally agreed consensus of safe levels of alcohol ingestion during pregnancy. Women are therefore encouraged to abstain from alcohol prior to and during pregnancy, or adhere to safety guidelines offered by the Royal College of Obstetricians and Gynaecologists (1995). Alcohol consumption may be linked with an increasing incidence of female infertility. High intakes of alcohol consumption (14 or more units per week), have been associated with reduced fecundability (the probability of achieving conception or a recognised pregnancy in a menstrual cycle). Several studies using retrospective data, however, identified no causal link between moderate alcohol consumption and reduced fecundability, which suggests that it is not a viable risk factor during the prenatal period (Olsen et al 1982, 1997). Jenson (1998) presents an opposing argument which suggests that alcoholic ingestion even at low levels reduces the chances of fertility. The study assessed the effects of moderate alcohol consumption on fecundability. Prospective data of 430 couples for six consecutive menstrual cycles (or until pregnancy was achieved) were collected. After adjustment for non-alcoholic variables, the probability of achieving conception in a menstrual cycle decreased with increasing alcohol intake, from 0.61 among women consuming one to five drinks per week to 0.34 among those taking 10 drinks per week (Jenson 1998). The researcher concluded that women should be discouraged from taking alcohol when they are trying to become pregnant.

Nutrition advice is essential when discussing alcohol consumption. Ethanol (present in alcohol) is a known source of energy, therefore, high alcohol levels may influence the desire to eat adequately. Alcohol has been shown to interfere with the absorption of many nutrients including intestinal absorption of calcium, amino acids and vitamins: thiamin, folate and vitamin K (Wardlow, Insel & Seyler 1997). It is suggested that women with a history of alcohol abuse must be given multivitamins, including folic acid, prenatally and throughout pregnancy (Bradley & Bennett 1997). The correlation between alcohol and sperm morphology is weak despite an association between regular drinking by the male and reduced birth weight of the infant. Irrespective of these findings, men should restrict their drinking 4 months prior to conception (Dunphy, Barratt & Cooke 1991, Parazzini et al 1993). (Ch. 7 offers a detailed approach to alcohol consumption during pregnancy.)

Drugs

Maternal and paternal drug abuse is fraught with problems. Significant evidence suggests that it may result in poor pregnancy outcome (Gilbert & Harman 1998, Queenan & Hobbins 1996). Counselling and advice should be offered, but referral to specialist support agencies is necessary. Detoxification and rehabilitation programmes may be viable referral options for those who feel able to make positive lifestyle choices and progress toward their ultimate aim of reproduction.

Environmental factors

Scientific evidence is gradually accumulating which associates environmental toxins with male and female infertility, miscarriage and fetal deformity

(Swan & Apgar 1995). Lead is a known toxin with accumulating levels adversely affecting health. It is predominantly found in lead petrol, foods grown from soil polluted by lead petrol and water from old lead piping (Ward 1987). It is suggested that cigarette smoking can increase lead uptake by 25%, partly because of its increased affinity and interaction with cigarette chemicals. High levels of lead exposure have a capacity for inducing abortions. A possible explanation is its readiness to accumulate in placental tissues at toxic levels (Bradley & Bennett 1997). Analysis of maternal and neonatal tissue, including placental material, has shown high levels of lead and cadmium and low levels of zinc which contribute to stillbirths and fetal malformations (Ward & Bryce-Smith 1993). Protection from occupational hazards, pesticides, lead, mercury and solvents is important. This includes utilisation of protective clothing in the home and the workplace where appropriate and adhering to safety parameters and work codes will minimise exposure to teratogenic toxins.

Social factors

Childbirth and parenting can have a profound impact on family systems. Discussion and exploration of expectations, social support systems and socioeconomic circumstances can facilitate forward thinking, preparation and planning. Identifying stressors is particularly important and may in turn identify coping behaviours, including smoking, drinking and/or illicit drug use. Problem and abusive relationships may also be identified. A study which sought to investigate whether maternal anxiety in the third trimester of pregnancy was associated with adverse fetal effect presented interesting findings. A mechanism by which the psychological state of the mother affects fetal development was identified and may explain the association between maternal anxiety and low birth weight (Teixeira, Fisk & Glove 1999). The midwife must be in a position to support, guide and counsel the woman and her partner, or refer them to an appropriate support group/agency where they may achieve the maximum amount of help and support to enable them to make an informed choice about future reproduction. Midwives may choose to explore reasons for the intended pregnancy and increase awareness of the impact pregnancy, childbirth and parenting may have on existing lifestyle. Williamson, LeFevre & Hector (1989) suggest that a progressive increase in stressful life change is associated with adverse outcome. Women who experienced increased psychosocial stress during the second and third trimester of pregnancy were significantly more likely to have babies with Apgar scores less than seven at 5 minutes, transfer to a neonatal intensive care unit and birth weight below 2.5 kg. Obstetric risk factors and demographic details were controlled for during the study.

Contraception

Establishing a woman's menstrual history is vitally important. Exploring her ideas about menstruation and ovulation may be a worthwhile trigger for education and discussion about achieving conception. It should not be assumed that all women are aware of how the menstrual cycle works. Menstrual dysfunction can be established only on this basis. Advice about current contraceptive use should include the effects of contraception on the ability to conceive; this may include advice, for example, on the contraceptive pill. The use of oral contraception has been found to be associated with vitamin and mineral imbalances. The pill has been found to raise copper and lower zinc levels in the body, leaving women who conceive after coming off the pill in a zinc deficient state. Zinc deficiency has been associated with postnatal depression and lactation problems. Excess copper has been associated with conditions including postnatal depression and pre-eclampsia (Bradley & Bennett 1997). This conclusion, however, is not supported by other research evidence. As a part of the preparation for pregnancy, it is essential that women stop oral contraception use, at least 6 months prior to pregnancy, so that the nutritional and hormonal states can be rebalanced to maintain a pregnancy successfully (Bradley & Bennett 1997).

Dietary factors

The aim of dietary advice is to ensure that an optimal nutritional state is achieved prior to conception. This has been thought to maximise the chances of conception and increase the chances of a healthy infant being born. Women who are obese should be referred for dietary advice (if the obesity is due to dietary factors) regarding preconception weight loss. The obese woman is at an increased risk of developing gestational diabetes (Blackburn & Loper 1992). Women who are sufferers of anorexia nervosa, or who are underweight, have a higher risk of fetal and neonatal death (Swan & Apgar 1995). Clear evidence has indicated that maternal malnutrition and suboptimal nutritional states adversely affect the health and future development of the fetus. There is some evidence to suggest that the effects of suboptimal nutrition are associated with low birth weight babies, who are programmed for the development of disorders later in life, including coronary heart disease and diabetes (Barker 1994). Further evidence shows that death from ischaemic heart disease and cerebrovascular accidents are significantly reduced with increasing birth weight (Leeson, Wincup & Cook 1997). It is clear that maternal nutrition has a profound effect on the pregnancy and the fetus. Increasing speculation will continue about the long term health effects, which may determine the patterns of health well into the 21st century. The body mass index (BMI) should be used when advising women about nutrition before conception. This is a reliable indicator to identify nutritional status (United States Institution of Medicine 1990). BMI is defined as the weight in kilograms divided by height in metres. It is suggested that fertility begins to decline as BMI falls below approximately 23 kg per metre. Preconception dietary counselling and advice may help underweight women progress toward a more favourable BMI. Accumulating evidence suggests that fasting for 1 day adversely affects hormone levels of progesterone and oestradiol the following night and therefore reduces the woman's chances of conception. If she does conceive, her chances of miscarriage are increased or she may be at an increased risk of having a low birth weight baby (Cooper et al 1995). Women should therefore be advised about the regularity of meals as well as the inadequacy (Wynn & Wynn 1995). The adequacy of the diet during pregnancy has received increasing attention. A study carried out by Wynn & Wynn (1994) sought to show the influence of a low calorie diet on the ability to ovulate in a subject who had previously had a normal diet and normal progesterone surge during the second half of the menstrual cycle (luteal phase). The subject was given a reducing diet of only 1000 calories per day beginning at the start of a menstrual cycle. Subsequently there was no ovulation and menstruation. No luteal phase progesterone surge was identified. Once the subject's normal diet was resumed, her fertility resumed. Although this study examines an individual case, the researchers propose that if the diet falls below a certain standard the endocrine systems do not function to promote fertility. General advice may be to eat to hunger and drink to thirst. The exceptions are for those who suffer from eating disorders such as anorexia, are alcohol dependent, and therefore rely on ethanol as sources of energy, or heavy cigarette smokers who have an appetite suppressant toward carbohydrates.

Clients who may benefit from individual counselling or referral to specialist agents where appropriate include:

- adolescent mothers who may have, for example, inadequate dietary intake due to body image dissatisfaction or lack of nutritional awareness
- low income groups who may overrely on high fat and sugar convenience foods
- vegetarians with inadequate diet (Ready, Sanders & Obeid 1994, Sanders & Reddy 1994)
- women with pre-existing medical conditions such as diabetes mellitus, cystic fibrosis or gastrointestinal problems (Thomas 1994).

Discussion with regards to a diet adequate in iron would be advisable as during pregnancy the increase in red cell volume demands an increase in iron. Vitamin C intake should also be discussed, in light of its necessity for iron absorption.

Vitamins

Nutritional requirements for vitamins and minerals are increased during pregnancy. It is suggested that the diets of those who live in industrialised countries contain a high proportion of refined foods and are therefore more likely to require vitamin supplementation (Bradley & Bennett 1997). Despite healthy-eating advice, the uptake of vitamin supplementation remains relatively low. A study describing the diet of 11 923 pregnant women concluded that the diets of pregnant women in England are likely to contain adequate amounts of most nutrients, the most likely exceptions being iron, magnesium, potassium and folate. At the time of the study all who took part had contact with a midwife and general practitioner and were at 32 weeks' gestation. The researchers expressed concern at the low levels of folate intake because of its association with neural tube defect (Rogers et al 1998). Midwives should continue to offer advice and guidance tailored to meet the individual needs of the client, in order to have maximum impact. Gillies & Spray (1997) suggest that interventions focused toward the individual which involve counselling, reinforcement, support, information, personal skills development and coping strategies encourage health-related behavioural change in up to one in four of those who participate.

Personal dietary needs are partly determined by lifestyle, habits, nutritional patterns and medical and reproductive history. Caution should be advised when vitamin A supplements are being taken, as a tentative link between excessive vitamin A intake and congenital abnormalities is still apparent. When advising women about supplementation, it is worthwhile discussing the source of vitamin A considered to be teratogenic to the fetus. Vitamin A can be consumed as preformed vitamin A (retinoids), found in animal sources, or the vitamin A precursor beta carotene (carotenoids), found in plant sources (green vegetables and fruit). The plant source is considered to be perfectly safe with no teratogenic effects on humans. However, extensive research evidence points to the teratogenic effects of retinoids on the fetus (Pinnock & Alderman 1992, Rothman et al 1995). Liver and liver products contain as much as 12 times the recommended daily amount of vitamin A. The recommended daily allowance is 400 IU; most antenatal vitamins contain 800 IU (Cefalo, Bowes & Moos 1995). Women who take more than the recommended daily requirement of vitamin A during pregnancy expose the infant to growth and developmental risk. The prevalence of cranial neural crest defects among offspring of women who took 10 000 IU/d of vitamin A supplementation was reported to be 1.18% (Rothman et al 1995). Women should be advised to avoid vitamin A supplementation and foods rich in vitamin A as high doses are teratogenic.

Vitamin D and calcium requirements are usually met by increased absorption from the gut during pregnancy to meet the demands of the growing fetus. When advising teenagers, however, it may be useful to discuss calcium and vitamin D requirements in further detail as bone growth may not be complete.

A diet balanced with the recommended daily requirements of vitamin E has been associated with prevention of miscarriage and with strengthening uterine muscles (Marks 1979, Williams 1973). This correlation, however, is weak and warrants further research.

Folic acid

Approximately 500 pregnancies a year are known to be affected by neural tube defect (Murphy et al 1996). It is now generally accepted that increased folate intake before and during early pregnancy reduces the occurrence and recurrence of neural tube defects, namely spina bifida, anencephaly and encephalocoele (Medical Research Council 1991). The DOH (1992b) has recommended that women take at least 400 µg of folic acid daily as a single preparation prior to conception and continue to do so during the first trimester of pregnancy. Overwhelming evidence has suggested that taking folic acid in this way can reduce the incidence of neural tube malformations by 72% (Medical Research Council 1991). The mechanism responsible is not clearly understood. Most studies have reported a protective effect of either dietary folate, folic acid supplements or multivitamin supplements containing folic acid (Czeizel & Dudas 1992, Werler, Shapiro & Mitchell 1993). When providing advice about the source of adequate folic acid intake, consideration of the following discussion is worthwhile. An ingestion of large volumes of multivitamins would be necessary in order to achieve the recommended daily requirement of folic acid and produce its protective effect. Other vitamin groups in the preparation would result in toxicity.

As humans cannot synthesise folates they are dependent on dietary sources. Encouraging women to increase their dietary folate as a means of protecting against the prevalence of neural tube defect may be misleading. Foods fortified with folic acid and synthetic folic acid in vitamin supplements are efficiently absorbed as they are present in a monoglutamate form, whereas folates naturally occurring in food are present in a polyglutamate form and require conversion to monoglutamates by intestinal enzymes prior to absorption (Czeizel 1995). Reider (1994) demonstrated that 90% of folate content of vitamin preparations are absorbed, as opposed to 50% of food folate polyglutamates. A research study which aimed to show that food fortification and vitamin supplementation are more efficient methods of increasing folate status than natural food folate demonstrated interesting results (Cuskelly, McNulty & Scott 1996). Women were randomly assigned to five groups, namely: folic acid supplementation, folic acid-fortified foods, dietary folate, dietary advice and a control group. All groups were followed over a 3 month period. Red cell folate concentrations increased significantly in the groups taking folic acid supplements and foods fortified with folic acid by the end of the 3 month period. In contrast, there was no significant change in folate status in groups which used dietary folate and dietary advice groups to raise folate levels. The researchers concluded that the most likely explanation for these findings is the increased availability of folic acid in the monoglutamate form as opposed to the polyglutamate form. Clinicians should still advise women to take foods rich in folate but emphasis should be placed on increasing the consumption of foods fortified with folic acid and folic acid supplements. One of the five campaign objectives agreed by the HEA (1996) during their 3 year folic acid health promotion initiative (see below) was to increase the availability and number of folic acid-fortified foods. To this end, 101 breakfast cereals were reported to be fortified with folic acid in July 1996; this figure rose to 112 in December 1997. The number of breads fortified with folic acid rose from five in December 1995 to 20 in December 1997 (HEA 1996).

The neural tube closes by the end of the seventh week after the last menstrual period. Many women at this stage may not realise that they are pregnant. Providing health education for women who are planning a pregnancy would exclude the large proportion of unplanned pregnancies, therefore a whole population approach is justified. Raising public awareness through media campaigns and primary health care teams with an emphasis on dietary sources of folate and foods fortified with folate in women of childbearing age would increase the potential of those entering pregnancy, albeit unplanned, with an enhanced folate intake. The overwhelming message would be to encourage all those planning a pregnancy to take the recommended daily dosage of folic acid as well as paying attention to dietary folate intake.

Uptake of folic acid: is the health message getting across?

In 1995 the DOH carried out research which found that very few women were taking folic acid either during the preconception period or during the first trimester of pregnancy as previously recommended. They therefore commissioned the HEA to raise awareness among women of childbearing age about the protective effects of folic acid. The programme was launched in 1996 and was successful largely because of partnerships with the voluntary sector, professional organisations and government departments.

More recently a contraceptive manufacturer added a paragraph to the leaflet enclosed in the contraceptive pill packet, informing users of the benefits of taking folic acid supplementation once oral contraceptive use has ceased (HEA 1998). This approach will undoubtedly help to raise public awareness. Education of both the public and health care providers has been shown to increase the awareness of folate supplementation prior to and during pregnancy but the uptake still remains relatively low (Clark & Fisk 1994). Preconception care provides an opportunity to raise awareness about the benefits of folic acid supplementation, but unless the vitamin becomes more available and accessible the potential to influence uptake is lost. It is available over the counter and on prescription from the general practitioner. Despite motivation and intent to obtain folic acid, social deprivation, poverty and social isolation are but a few factors that would inhibit uptake. Individuals who are socioeconomically disadvantaged are more likely to be focusing energy and time toward managing a low income and coping with unemployment and poor housing, as opposed to attending the chemist or the general practitioner's surgery for folic acid tablets. During the HEA folic acid campaign, prescription rates for folic acid increased but the uptake in the socioeconomic disadvantaged groups remained significantly low. When counselling women about increasing their intake of folate, midwives should tailor their discussion toward the adoption of strategies which may prove successful. This will be possible for those who book early for antenatal care (see Box 5.1) or attend preconception care. Encouraging the uptake of bread fortified with folic acid as opposed to the more expensive food types may ensure successful uptake. Awareness of the negative effects of alcohol and smoking on the folate status is essential when providing health education advice. Piyathilake et al (1994) stated that smokers required an average folate intake of 658 µg per day to achieve a serum folate level equivalent to that of a non-smoker consuming 200 µg a day. Women who are prone to gastrointestinal disorders need specific advice as folic acid is predominantly absorbed in the duodenum and jejunum and as such metabolism and absorption may be inhibited (Czeizel 1995, Hine 1993). Women who are taking anticonvulsants, antacids and H_2 blockers prenatally require medical advice as these are known folate antagonists (Hine 1996). Overambitious attempts to increase folate intake above and beyond the recommended daily allowance should be discouraged. Large doses have been found to interfere with the diagnosis of pernicious anaemia.

Infection history

As the prevalence of HIV infection in women of reproductive age continues to rise, health professionals should ensure that all women planning a pregnancy are informed about the potential benefits of knowing their HIV infection status. There have been in excess of 4000 reports of HIV infection in women in the United Kingdom (Public Health Laboratory Service AIDS and STD Centre 1997), although anonymous testing reveals that this figure is grossly underestimated (Nicoll, McGarrigle & Brady 1998). It is vital that screening for HIV infection is discussed as part of preconception care. Establishing a woman's HIV status before pregnancy can enable her to make informed choices about becoming pregnant and inform her of the risks to herself and her unborn baby if she chose to become pregnant. Women who are found to be HIV seropositive will have the opportunity to be given accurate information on the risks of transmission and interventions available to reduce the risk to the baby, if the woman decided that pregnancy was still an option. Information and discussion points may be raised from the following;

• The rate of mother to child transmission in the United Kingdom and the rest of Europe is estimated to be 15 and 20% respectively, in non-breast feeding women who have no drug therapy (Peckham & Gibb 1995).
• To prevent perinatal transmission of HIV, women are now receiving antiretroviral therapy prior to pregnancy (Centres for Disease Control and Prevention 1998).
• Women who take zidovudine during the antenatal period reduce the transmission rates to approximately 5% (Fowler & Mofenson 1997, Mofenson 1997).
• Breast feeding doubles the rate of transmission (Peckham & Gibb 1995). During the postnatal period transmission can be reduced by half by avoiding breast feeding (Dunn et al 1992).
• Generally insurance companies are not concerned with negative tests. The Association of British Insurers (ABI 1997) 'no longer ask whether the applicant has had a test or counselling but confine questions to asking only about positive results and treatment'.

Screening for infections such as rubella and hepatitis prevent the huge emotional and financial consequence experienced if exposure takes place. Vaccines are readily available, and family-planning advice should be offered prior to giving the rubella vaccine. Rubella infection during the first trimester of pregnancy produces a fetal anomaly rate of 50% and in the second trimester 35%. Infection during the third trimester is reported to cause no adverse fetal harm. Infants born of mothers who are positive for hepatitis B surface antigen or hepatitis B 'e' antigen are suggested to have a 70–90% chance of acquiring perinatal hepatitis; therefore preparation and early vaccination are essential (Stevens et al 1985). Screening for sexually transmitted diseases, including genital herpes simplex virus, chlamydial infections and human papillomavirus, should be an integral part of the screening programme. Screening for tuberculosis, toxoplasmosis and cytomegalovirus may be carried out if exposure has been likely. Adequate education and preparation should be offered prior to screening procedures to enable women and their partners, if present, to make informed decisions.

Previous obstetric history

Discussion of previous obstetric history may prompt the disclosure of abnormal events previously perceived to be normal, particularly when the outcome was positive.

Detailed information about all aspects of the pregnancy, labour and the puerperium should be sought and recorded. This forum may be used by the client as an opportunity to discuss previous birth outcomes where fears and anxieties have not been resolved.

Medical factors

Identification of medical or surgical factors which may influence fertilisation, conception, maintenance of pregnancy and pregnancy outcome can provide an opportunity during preconception care for education, counselling and possible referral to specialist agencies. Clients can therefore have appropriate time to make informed decisions about future reproduction. Conditions which may necessitate genetic enquiry include:

- Tay–Sachs disease
- beta thalassaemia
- alpha thalassaemia
- sickle cell anaemia
- cystic fibrosis or fragile X or Down's syndrome.

Epilepsy

During the preconception period antiepileptic drugs should be evaluated for their need, the minimum dose required to prevent seizures and their potential harm to the fetus (Queenan & Hobbins 1996). The adverse effects of seizures on pregnancy are likely to be greater if anticonvulsants are not used (Cefalo, Bowes & Moos 1995). Education regarding the teratogenic effects of specific anticonvulsants can be discussed during consultation with the neurologist to develop an individualised drug regimen that balances maternal seizure control with fetal side-effects.

Phenylketonuria

Women who have phenylketonuria and have blood phenylalanine levels of 20 mg/dl have an increased risk of having infants who have microcephaly, mental retardation, congenital heart disease and intrauterine growth retardation (Platt, Koch & Azen 1992). Preconception care would involve working toward achieving a blood phenylalanine level that protected the fetus against the effects, which is suggested to be around 10 mg/dl. Dietary advice and support would be essential to ensure maintenance throughout pregnancy.

Diabetes mellitus

Due to the availability of insulin, women with diabetes are able to conceive and produce healthy offspring. Prior to the 1920s, when insulin was not available, conception and the maintenance of a pregnancy was a remote possibility. Pregnancy is a diabetogenic state characterised by mild fasting hypoglycaemia, postprandial hypoglycaemia and hyperinsulinaemia. Such changes occur to ensure that the fetus receives adequate glucose levels. Pregnancy therefore affects the already altered metabolism (Queenan & Hobbins 1996). Preconception care of the diabetic client can provide a forum where stressing the importance of glucose control forms an integral part of education and counselling. Gabbe (1996) suggests that if glucose is adequately controlled before and during pregnancy the fetal survival rate is approximated to be 95 to 97%. The aim of care would be to assess glycaemic control and stress the importance of maintaining control so as to achieve maximum fertility and optimum embryonic and fetal growth. This would minimise the risk of spontaneous abortion, pre-eclampsia, preterm labour, polyhydramnios, infection, congenital malformations, macrosomia, intrauterine growth retardation and neonatal hyper- and hypoglycaemia (American College of Obstetrics and Gynecology (ACOG) 1994). Clients may be advised to seek advice from their general practitioners who may also refer them on for dietetic advice. (See recommended reading list as a reference point for more information.)

Summary

- The preconception period is an extremely important time where conditions for reproduction must be optimised in order for conception to occur and embryonic development to progress without adverse outcome.
- The midwife is the ideal health professional to provide preconception care. The obvious benefits with regards to continuity are unquestionable. Unfortunately, due to reduced resource commitment and financial allocation, the current provision of care is sparse.
- The focus of health promotion during the preconception period has the potential to increase the chances of conception and maintenance of pregnancy whilst optimising the pregnancy outcome with minimal risks to the mother and the fetus.
- Preconception care counselling involves identifying potential risk factors and discussing strategies to decrease or remove the risk. Counselling and advice about, for example, exercise and diet, environmental poisons and social poisons, smoking cessation and alcohol abuse programmes can have positive effects on health gain and long term social and financial benefits.
- It is important for clinicians involved in providing preconception care to keep up to date with resources that are shown through research to

be effective in rehabilitating, ameliorating or promoting healthy lifestyle choices.

- It is only with accumulating evidence of cost/benefit of preconception care health gain that health care services will take the need for preconception care programmes seriously.
- Setting up of a preconception clinic requires an enormous amount of time resources and financial commitment, not to mention the additional training of staff in subjects including nutrition, mineral metabolism, allergy and environmental toxins.
- Raising awareness about the male influence on a successful pregnancy and also the supportive role in relation to lifestyle modification is invaluable. However, until routine preconception care is available to all women and their partners many opportunities for the primary prevention of poor reproductive outcomes will be lost.
- Lack of preconception care or awareness of health risks is a lost opportunity for women to modify behaviours that may adversely affect the course and outcome of pregnancy.
- All women have the right to be given information which could adversely influence their reproductive futures. Given the high proportion of unplanned pregnancies, primary prevention strategies for birth defects must involve all women of childbearing age, not simply those planning a pregnancy.
- Although public health initiatives have had a huge impact on the population's health over the last century, a more specific approach and commitment from government should be presented to enable preconception care to be widely available and taken more seriously.

References

American College of Obstetrics and Gynecology (ACOG) 1994 Diabetes and pregnancy. ACOG technical bulletin no 200, December

Association of British Insurers 1997 ABI Statement of practice – underwriting life insurance for HIV/AIDS. Association of British Insurers, London

Atik R B 1994 Statistics on miscarriage. Miscarriage Association, Wakefield, Yorks

Barker D J B 1994 Mothers, babies and disease in later life. BMJ Publications, London

Blackburn S, Loper D 1992 Maternal, fetal and neonatal physiology: a clinical perspective. W B Saunders, Philadelphia

Bradley S, Bennett N 1997 Preparation for pregnancy: an essential guide. Argyll, Glendaruel, Scotland

Cefalo R, Moos M 1988 Preconceptional health promotion: a practical guide. Aspen, Rockville MD

Cefalo R, Bowes W, Moos M 1995 Preconception care: a means of prevention. Baillière's Clinical Obstetrics and Gynaecology 9(3):403–416

Centres for Disease Control and Prevention 1998 Administration of zidovudine during late pregnancy and delivery to prevent perinatal HIV transmission – Thailand 1996–1998. Morbidity and Mortality Weekly Report 47:151–154

Chamberlain G 1980 The prepregnancy clinic. British Medical Journal 281:31–35

Chapple 1991 House of Commons Health Committee fourth report maternity services: preconception, vol 1. HMSO, London

Clark N A C, Fisk N M 1994 Minimal compliance with the Department of Health recommendation for routine folate prophylaxis to prevent neural tube defects. British Journal of Obstetrics and Gynaecology 101:709–710

Cooper R L, DuBard M B, Golenburg R L, Oweis A I 1995 The relationship of maternal attitude toward weight gain during pregnancy and low birth weight. Obstetrics and Gynaecology 85(4):591–595

Cuskelly G J, McNulty H, Scott J M 1996 Effect of increasing dietary folate on red-cell folate: implications for prevention of neural tube defects. Lancet 347:657–659

Czeizel A E 1995 Folic acid in the prevention of neural tube defects. Journal of Pediatric Gastroenterology and Nutrition 20(1):4–16

Czeizel A E, Dudas I 1992 Prevention of first occurrence of neural tube defects by periconceptional vitamin supplementation. New England Journal of Medicine 327:1832–1835

Department of Health (DOH) 1992a The health of the nation. Eat well: action plan from the Nutrition Task Force. DOH, London

Department of Health (DOH) 1992b Folic acid and the prevention of neural tube defects. Report from an expert advisory group. DOH, London

Dunkley J 1997 Training midwives to help pregnant women stop smoking. Nursing Times 93(5):64–66

Dunn D, Newell M L, Ades A, Peckham C 1992 Risk of human immunodeficiency virus type 1 transmission through breast feeding. Lancet 340:585–588

Dunphy B C, Barratt C L R, Cooke I D 1991 Male alcohol consumption and fecundity in couples attending an infertility clinic. Andrologia 23:219–221

Fowler M G, Mofenson L 1997 Progress in prevention of perinatal HIV-1. Acta Paediatrica (suppl) 421:97–106

Gabbe S 1996 Diabetes mellitus. In: Queenan J, Hobbins J (eds) Protocols for high risk pregnancies, 3rd edn. Blackwell Science, Cambridge, England

Gilbert E S, Harman J S 1998 High risk pregnancy and delivery, 2nd edn. Mosby, New York

Gillies P, Spray J 1997 Addressing health inequalities: the practical potential of social capital. Health Education Authority, London

Hawkes N 1994 Babies may be paying a high price for grandmother's habit. The Times (3 February):78–80

Health Education Authority (HEA) 1996 Folic acid campaign, local activity handbook. HEA, London

Health Education Authority (HEA) 1998 Contraceptives to include folic acid (news release). HEA, London

Hellerstedt W, Pirie P, Lando H, Curry S, McBride C, Grothaus L, Nelson J 1998 Differences in preconceptional and prenatal behaviours in women with intended and unintended pregnancies. American Journal of Public Health 88(4):663–666

Hine J 1993 Folic acid: contemporary clinical perspective. Perspectives in Applied Nutrition 1(2):3–13

Hine R J 1996 What practitioners need to know about folic acid. Journal of the American Dietician Association 86(5):451–453

House of Commons Health Committee 1991 Fourth report maternity services: preconception, vol 1. Report with proceedings of the Health Committee. HMSO, London

Jack B, Culpepper L 1990 Preconception care. In: Merkatz I R, Thompson J E (eds) New perspectives on prenatal care. Elsevier, New York, pp 70–78

Jenson T K 1998 Alcohol ante/postnatal care. British Medical Journal 317:505–510

Kings Fund Centre 1992 A positive approach to nutrition as treatment. Kings Fund, London

Leeson C P M, Wincup P H, Cook D G 1997 Flow-mediated dilatation in nine to eleven year old children. Circulation 96(7):233–237

Marks J 1979 A guide to the vitamins. Medical and Technical Publishers, Lancaster

Marsack C, Alsop C, Kurinczuk J, Bower C 1995 Pre-pregnancy counselling for the primary prevention of birth defects: rubella vaccination and folate intake. Medical Journal of Australia 162:403–406

Medical Research Council Vitamin Study Research Group 1991 Prevention of neural tube defects, results of the medical research council vitamin study. Lancet 338:131–137

Mofenson L M 1997 Interaction between timing of potential human immunodeficiency virus infection and the design of preventive and therapeutic interventions. Acta Paediatrica (suppl) 421:1–9

Mulliner C M 1995 A study exploring midwives' education in knowledge of and attitudes towards nutrition in pregnancy. Midwifery 11(1):37–41

Murphy M, Seagroatt V, Hey K et al 1996 Neural tube defects 1974–1994 – down but not out. Archives of Disease in Childhood 75:F133–134

Nicoll A, McGarrigle C, Brady T 1998 Epidemiology and detection of HIV-1 among pregnant women in the United Kingdom: results from national surveillance 1988–1996. British Medical Journal 316:253–258

Office for National Statistics 1997 Government statistical service. Mortality statistics – childhood, infant and perinatology, England and Wales (series DH3 no 28) 1997. The Stationery Office, London

Olsen J, Rachootin P, Schiedt A V, Damsbo N 1982 Tobacco use, alcohol consumption and infertility. International Journal of Epidemiology 12:179–184

Olsen J, Bolumar F, Boldsen J, Bisanti L 1997 The European Study Group of infertility and subfecundity. Does moderate alcohol intake reduce fecundability? A European multicentre study on infertility and subfecundity. Alcoholism, Clinical and Experimental Research 21:206–212

Parazzini F, Marchini M, Tozzi L et al 1993 Risk factors for unexplained dyspermia in infertile men. A case-control study. Archives of Andrology 31:105–113

Peckham C S, Gibb D 1995 Mother to child transmission of the human immunodeficiency virus. New England Journal of Medicine 333:298–302

Pinnock C B, Alderman C P 1992 The potential for teratogenicity of vitamin A and its congeners. Medical Journal of Australia 22:66–70

Piyathilake C J, Macaluso M, Hine R J et al 1994 Local and systematic effects of cigarette smoking on folate and vitamin B12. American Journal of Clinical Nutrition 60:559–566

Platt L D, Koch R, Azen C 1992 Maternal phenylketonuria collaborative study, obstetrics aspect and outcome: the first six years. American Journal of Obstetrics and Gynecology 166:1150–1162

Public Health Laboratory Service AIDS and STD Centre – Communicable Disease Surveillance Centre and Scottish Centre for Infection and Environmental Health 1997 Quarterly surveillance tables 38, data to the end of December 1997

Queenan J, Hobbins J 1996 Protocols for high risk pregnancies. Blackwell Science, New York

Ready S, Sanders T A B, Obeid O 1994 The influence of maternal vegetarian diet on essential fatty acid status of the new-born. European Journal of Clinical Nutrition (48)5:358–368

Reider M J 1994 Prevention of neural tube defects with periconceptual folic acid. Clinical Perinatology 21(3):483–503

Rogers I, Emmett P, the ALSPAC study team 1998 Diet during pregnancy in a population of pregnant women in South West England. European Journal of Clinical Nutrition 58:246–250

Rothman K J, Moore L L, Singer M R, Nguyen U, Mannino S, Milunsky A 1995 Teratogenicity of high vitamin A intake. New England Journal of Medicine 333(21):1369–1373

Royal College of Obstetricians and Gynaecologists (RCOG) 1995 Alcohol consumption in pregnancy guideline. RCOG 9:1–4

Sanders T A B, Reddy S 1994 Vegetarian diets and children. American Journal of Clinical Nutrition 59 (suppl):1176S–1181S

Secretary of State for Health 1998 Our healthier nation, a contract for health. A consultation paper. The Stationery Office, London

Stevens C E, Toy P T, Tong M J et al 1985 Perinatal hepatitis B virus transmission in the United States. Prevention by passive-active immunisation. Journal of the American Medical Association 253:1740–1745

Swan L, Apgar B 1995 Preconceptual obstetric risk assessment and health promotion. American Family Physician 51(8):1807–1885

Teixeira J M A, Fisk N M, Glove V 1999 Association between maternal anxiety in pregnancy and increased uterine artery resistance index: cohort based study. British Medical Journal 318:153–157

Thomas 1994 The manual of dietetic practice, 2nd edn. Blackwell Scientific, London

United States Institution of Medicine 1990 Nutrition during pregnancy. National Academy Press, Washington DC

Wallace M, Hurwitz B 1998 Preconception care: who needs it, who wants it, and how should it be provided? British Journal of General Practice 48 (February):963–966

Ward N 1987 Placental element levels in relation to fetal development for obstetrically 'normal' births: a study of 37 elements, evidence for effects of cadmium, lead and zinc on fetal growth and smoking as a source of cadmium. International Journal of Biosocial Research 9(1):63

Ward N I, Bryce-Smith D 1993 Lead, cadmium and zinc levels in relation to fetal development and abnormalities. In: Allan R J, Nriagu J O (eds) Heavy metals in the environment, vol 2. CEP Consultants, Edinburgh, pp 280–284

Wardlow G, Insel P, Seyler M 1997 Contemporary nutrition: issues and insights, 2nd edn. Mosby, St Louis

Werler M, Shapiro S, Mitchell A 1993 Periconceptional folic acid exposure and risk of occurrent neural tube defects. Journal of the American Medical Association 269:1257–1261

Williams R 1973 Nutrition against disease. Bantam, London

Williamson H A, LeFevre M, Hector M 1989 Association between life stress and serious perinatal complications. Journal of the Family Practitioner 29(5):489–494

Wynn M, Wynn A 1994 Slimming and fertility. Modern Midwife (June):17–20

Wynn M, Wynn A 1995 A fertility diet for planning pregnancy. Nutrition and Health 10:219–238

Recommended reading

American Diabetes Association 1998 Report of the expert committee on the diagnosis and classification of diabetes mellitus (committee report). Diabetes Care 21 (suppl 1):S5–S19

Bradley S G, Bennett N 1997 Preparation for pregnancy: an essential guide. Argyll Publishing, Glendaruel, Scotland
A guide to preconception care, with benefits of providing the service clearly demonstrated.

Harper P S 1993 Practical genetic counselling, 4th edn. Butterworth-Heinemann, Oxford

Health Education Authority (HEA) 1997a Folic acid and folates: tracking survey among women aged 16–45. HEA, London

Health Education Authority (HEA) 1997b and BMRB International. Folic acid and folates: tracking survey among women aged 16–45. HEA, London

Institute of Medicine, Food and Nutrition Board 1990 Subcommittee on nutrition status and weight gain during pregnancy: nutrition during pregnancy. weight gain. National Academy Press, Washington DC

Kitzmiller J L, Buchanan T A, Kjos S, Combs C A, Ratner R 1996 Preconception care of diabetes, congenital malformations, and spontaneous abortions (technical review). Diabetes Care 19:514–541

6 Smoking during pregnancy – strategies for damage limitation

Key themes

- Government commitment to reduce the prevalence of smoking during pregnancy
- Smoking cessation intervention programmes
- Nicotine replacement therapy during pregnancy
- Why women smoke
- Risks of smoking during pregnancy, maternal and fetal
- Infants of families who smoke
- The midwife's role in identifying and supporting pregnant smokers who wish to quit or who wish to continue smoking throughout the pregnancy
- Challenging misconceptions

Overview

Smoking is reducing the female advantage in life expectancy and widening the social class divide in mortality (Callum 1998). Smoking by mothers during pregnancy and the postnatal period carries health risks for both the mothers and their babies. Twenty-four per cent of women smoke during pregnancy and only 33% of these give up whilst pregnant (Foster, Lader & Cheesbrough 1997).

Over the last decade we have gained momentum in developing skills to help those pregnant women who wish to give up smoking to do so successfully. We have also encouraged those who do not wish to give up smoking to participate in damage limitation, thereby reducing the ill effects of sidestream smoke to other family members. As suggested in previous chapters, pregnancy may be the only time in a woman's life where she is in regular contact with a health professional whose primary focus is to encourage or maintain health-enhancing behaviour for the woman and her family. Pregnancy is considered an ideal time to help women who wish to give up smoking to do so successfully. Women and their partners are often keen to make lifestyle changes which may benefit the health of their baby. The preconception period would be the ideal time for this change; however, this service is not readily available or accessible. Evidence suggests that prenatal intervention involving 10 minutes of counselling with aids to cessation, specifically designed for pregnant women, can double quit rates (University of York 1998).

It is the aim of this chapter to explore reasons why women smoke and discuss intervention programmes which have been successful in reducing the prevalence of smoking. Fetal risk and damage limitation will also be explored in the light of research-based evidence. The chapter is concluded by proposing a model of behavioural change which is easily utilised during health promotion work to aid smoking cessation or damage limitation.

Prior knowledge of the following areas will enable the reader to understand the issues discussed in this chapter more fully:

- the harmful effects of cigarette smoke
- the chemicals contained in cigarettes
- the effects of smoking during pregnancy on fetal development.

A commitment from the government

Our healthier nation, a consultation document on public health, proposed national contracts in four areas including heart disease, stroke and cancer, with a heavy focus on tobacco control measures (Secretary of State for Health 1998a). The consultation document made reference to a specific white paper which would detail government commitment towards helping people quit and reducing the prevalence of those who start. Smoking kills, a government white paper on tobacco, was thus published (Secretary of State for Health 1998b), and makes specific reference to ending tobacco advertising on billboards and in the printed media, in the press and through sponsorship. All directives should be adopted by 2006. The white paper proposes that tackling smoking is central to improving health in Britain and pledged funding of approximately £60 million toward delivering expert help to those most in need.

Smoking cessation intervention programmes

It is difficult to assess the nature of information women are given by midwives about smoking cessation and intervention techniques and even harder to assess the effectiveness of the intervention since this is not routinely measured. Relatively few studies have been undertaken which assess the effectiveness of midwives' smoking cessation interventions with women. Pregnant women cite health care providers as the most important source of information about health behaviour in pregnancy (Aaronson, Mural & Pfoutz 1988). Despite their potential impact, the evidence indicates that health care providers do not routinely provide smoking cessation interventions to pregnant smokers (Walsh & Redman 1993). Studies to date support the conclusion that higher antenatal quit rates can be achieved through intervention.

The intervention used by Svanberg (1992) involved giving women self-help manuals especially written for pregnant women on smoking cessation, followed by interviews with midwives. The intervention was compared with a control group who were given a basic fact sheet about smoking and pregnancy and a recommendation to stop smoking. The study found that more women stopped smoking in the treatment group than in the control group at 8 weeks' postpartum, and demonstrated a quit rate of 10% in the treatment group. The researcher suggests that with intense intervention methods the results may have been improved. Similarly a study using intervention methods which included client-centred counselling, continuity of the counselling relationship by the lead professional and smoking cessation support aids was carried out. This study demonstrated quit rates of 9% in the treatment group and no behaviour change in the control group ($P > 0.05$). The intervention began after the booking interview, at 17 weeks' gestation (Dunkley 1997). The researcher suggests that women are more likely to change their smoking behaviour once they become pregnant or during the first trimester. They are more receptive to change at this time.

A trial of health education aimed at reducing cigarette smoking among pregnant women was reported by Rush et al (1992). The intervention used to influence smoking behaviour was counselling, which began at the first antenatal visit and continued throughout pregnancy. Reported quit rates were 10.4% in the treatment group and 5.4% in the control group. The results were not statistically significant. Counselling alone was therefore not successful in producing significant results.

Arborelius, Krakau & Bremberg (1992) aimed to design an effective course in helping pregnant women stop smoking. General practitioners and general nurses at two health care centres were interviewed. The aim was to establish procedure and perceived barriers to prevention, prior to the development of the programme. The results demonstrated that most doctors and nurses regarded health counselling as important in the medical health service. They also maintained that they had time and space for this activity. However, most doctors and nurses were hesitant and/or disappointed concerning their perceived efficacy in affecting people's life habits. An explanation offered by the researchers was that many doctors and nurses had a non-patient-centred style, which previous studies had demonstrated to be less successful in affecting people's behaviour. The results demonstrated the need for a client-centred approach to counselling. Wilms & Best (1991) emphasised the importance of the client's own decision in changing such life habits. The results of a study which shared similar aims showed that 88% of midwives felt that they played a significant role in helping pregnant women stop smoking, but 65% felt that they needed further training in smoking cessation and intervention techniques (Dunkley, unpublished research 1997). Recommendations for health commissioners outlined in the Smoking cessation guidelines for health professionals (HEA 1999) identify the need for core funding to integrate smoking cessation into health services and existing training budgets to prioritise smoking cessation training.

Mass media campaigns have been used as an intervention method to help reduce the prevalence of smoking. This method warrants further research in bringing the benefits of health promotion to deprived areas. Flay et al (1993) state that it is difficult to design mass media health promotion campaigns that bring about meaningful behaviour change in a large population of exposed persons. Televised smoking cessation clinics typically help only 4 to 5% of smokers to quit and maintain this for approximately 1 year. Supplementing the clinics with written material may double the effectiveness. Media programmes have low success rates for many reasons, including not reaching the target audience enough times, not gaining the attention of the target audience even when it is reached, using messages that are not fully comprehensible to it and using ineffective messages (Chapman & Egger 1993). Newspapers, occasional television programmes, women's magazines, leaflets and government health warnings on cigarettes and some cigarette advertisements warn pregnant mothers of the negative consequences of smoking on the health of the unborn child. This approach to health education is based on the belief that any change in the patterns of an individual's behaviour is the outcome of a triadic sequence: knowledge gained (1), leads to attitudinal change (2), which leads to behaviour being altered appropriately (3). However, information given in this way may have little effect on behavioural change but simply add additional guilt and anxiety. People motivated to change often do so independently of exposure to a televised programme on the topic. Although exposure to health warnings through television, leaflets and self-help manuals has had some success in helping pregnant women to stop smoking, face to face counselling is the most effective means of delivering anti-smoking messages (Dunkley 1997).

It is possible to alter smoking behaviour during pregnancy in a small minority of continuing smokers by a variety of strategies. Long term follow-up would give indication of prolonged success. Health professionals who have been given further training in smoking cessation and intervention skills are more likely to intervene and support smokers than those who have not been given further training. Silagy et al (1998a) suggest that smokers are more likely to stop if they have been supported by a health professional trained specifically in smoking cessation and intervention techniques.

Recently, evidence-based guidelines for smoking cessation issued by the HEA (1999) recommended that pregnant smokers should be given clear advice to stop smoking throughout pregnancy, and given the assistance when it is requested. They also recommend that 10 minutes or more of counselling interaction, supplemented by self-help materials, is an effective intervention for smoking cessation. This method of counselling shows an approximate doubling of cessation from about 8% (with usual care practices) to about 15% (Fiore et al 1996).

It is evident that no single method of intervention will help women to quit smoking successfully during pregnancy. It can be concluded that smoking cessation counselling is not yet integrated into routine practice. If service delivery is to improve, rigorous evaluation should be carried out to determine the effectiveness of the intervention and an assessment of costs involved. There is definitely a need for more research to be carried out on the effectiveness of midwives providing smoking cessation interventions because of their wide access to smokers.

Nicotine replacement therapy

Nicotine replacement therapy (NRT) has been utilised for non-pregnant smokers with increasing success (Fiore et al 1996, Silagy et al 1998b). Its use in pregnancy, however, remains contraindicated. Benowitz (1991) suggests that the benefits of NRT outweigh the risks of smoking for pregnant smokers, but suggests that NRT should be used only in extreme cases where the woman is a heavy smoker and cannot stop. Similarly, the American Agency for Health Care Policy and Research advocates the same approach for heavy pregnant smokers (Fiore et al 1996). The report of the Scientific Committee on Tobacco and Health recommended that research should be conducted into the efficacy and safety of NRT for pregnant smokers prior to its use (Poswillo 1998).

Understanding why women smoke

Understanding why women smoke can assist midwives in fine tuning their counselling to meet women's needs. Some practitioners still remain sceptical and pessimistic about the pregnant woman's ability to stop smoking during what is considered to be a time of considerable change and adaptation to pregnancy and motherhood. Other barriers to health promotion work in this area include lack of time, lack of skills and the perception of low success rates (Owen & Scott 1995). Midwives should regard smoking cessation and intervention techniques as an integral part of their role. Education and resource allocation will enable midwives to possess the confidence and skills necessary to interact effectively with women and their partners. Resources, time and commitment should be available for the service provision and there should be support from peers, superiors and professional bodies (Walsh & Redman 1993).

As stated previously, there are many studies which have attempted to demonstrate the need for a more timely and appropriate intervention approach to smoking cessation. Studies have consistently reported increased quit rates among women during early pregnancy although a substantial proportion of pregnant women continue to smoke (HEA 1999). Smoking during pregnancy does not appear to result from ignorance of the possible harmful effects, since the majority of women who continue to smoke during pregnancy know the basic hazards. Intervention strategies that rely heavily on information about the detrimental effects of cigarette smoke on the fetus will not have the desired effect. Women who are socioeconomically disadvantaged are more likely to continue to smoke during pregnancy (Marsh & Mackay 1994). Although the addictive nature of nicotine is acknowledged and well cited as one of the reasons why people are unable to give up smoking, other factors should be taken into account. Smoking is often used as a coping strategy for stressful life circumstances. Encouraging smoking cessation without addressing socioeconomic disadvantage is counterproductive.

The trend of teenage smoking rates shows a significant increase in smoking among teenage girls (Diamond & Goddard 1995). In 1988, one in five 15 year olds smoked regularly, currently (1999) this figure is one in three. A recent study which sought to influence the uptake of smoking among teenagers demonstrated interesting findings. Interventions which progressed beyond giving information and included personal skills development was found to delay the onset of smoking for up to 5 or 6 years (Gordon 1997). Teenagers would therefore spend more of their youth without the harmful effects of cigarette smoke. Teenagers who smoke are more likely to continue to smoke through to adulthood. The earlier they start smoking the more likely they are to smoke for longer.

A major study by Marsh & Mackay (1994) found that women living on low incomes in Britain are more likely to start smoking and least able to afford it. They were also suggested to be more likely to suffer hardship because of their expenditure on tobacco.

Graham & Hunt (1998) found that cigarettes were used as cues for rest and relaxation periods during the day and they marked a time to be spent with adult friends as opposed to being with the children. These findings reinforce the notion that smoking can provide a mechanism for coping in

Discussion questions

- Within the current time constraints of antenatal appointments, how can midwives apply appropriate health promotion strategies to reduce the effects of cigarette smoke to the woman, fetus and significant others?

- Which smoking cessation intervention have you used, or observed being used?

- How successful was the intervention in terms of smoking cessation, reducing the number of cigarettes smoked and damage limitation?

everyday situations. The place of smoking in the lives of women in low income households has been found to be a priority area. It is clear that in low income households, where luxury items and leisure activities are given up to make ends meet, cigarettes may be the only purchase a woman can make for personal enjoyment and relaxation. Most women smoke to control their levels of relaxation, pleasure, boredom or to 'calm their nerves' (Graham 1993, Greaves 1996). Health promotion interventions can be effective only if they are tailored to meet the individual needs of the client. Pregnant woman who live on low incomes and smoke cannot be cajoled into adopting a healthy lifestyle. Chapter 4 highlighted the complexities of behavioural change theory, the principles of which can be utilised to adopt the appropriate health promotion approach. Empowerment strategies and facilitating the development of social support may be a useful approach. The ultimate aim would be to enable women to develop alternative strategies for coping if they choose to stop smoking, and utilise the principles of damage limitation if they choose to continue. Self-efficacy would be an integral developmental part of this process. Graham & Hunt (1998) state that health promotion strategies aimed at reducing the pressures which smoking is seen to relieve is an effective approach to facilitating smoking cessation.

Risks of smoking

Maternal risks

Smoking during pregnancy is not without risk to the woman and the progress of pregnancy. Complications during pregnancy include:

- preterm labour (Lambers & Clark 1996)
- premature rupture of membranes (Andres 1996)
- spontaneous abortion (Fried 1993, Haglund & Cnattinguis 1990)
- placenta praevia (Andres 1996)
- abruptio placenta (Blackburn & Loper 1992)
- low birth weight (Fried 1993, Peacock, Bland & Anderson 1991).

Fetal risks

Cigarette smoking during pregnancy is a well-recognised health problem associated with several fetal and neonatal risks. Each cigarette contains over 2500 poisonous compounds, the effects of which are injurious to health. Carbon monoxide freely crosses the placenta and decreases the oxygen carrying capacity of the haemoglobin. Nicotine stimulates adrenergic release causing generalised vasoconstriction, leading to decreased uterine perfusion and narrowing of the umbilical arteries. Rises in the maternal and fetal heart rate and increased fetal movements are a compensatory response (ACOG 1993).

• Smoking during pregnancy has been found to be a contributory factor to intrauterine growth retardation.

• The association between smoking and average gestational age in some studies is weak (Backe 1993), although others suggest that the effect is dose dependent and is not the result of a shortened gestation period. Typically, infants of regular smokers are reported to weigh 150–250 g less than those of non-smokers (Secretary of State for Health 1998b).

• New evidence suggests that women who smoke during pregnancy pass harmful carcinogens on to their baby (Hecht et al 1998).

• Some studies have reported a significant relationship between lowered birth weight and the amount of secondhand smoke to which the pregnant non-smoker may be subjected (Mathai et al 1992). The concentrations of carbon monoxide and nicotine are approximately 2.5-fold higher in sidestream than in mainstream smoke (Mathai et al 1992). Passive smoking carries a health risk; this is clearly demonstrated by research showing that people who live or work in extremely smoky environments for long periods of time are 20% more likely to get cancer than are non-smokers (Hackshaw, Law & Wald 1997). From analysis of epidemiological studies it is suggested that maternal smoking in pregnancy is associated with a significant increase in the incidence of premature rupture of membranes and preterm labour. The precise biochemical mechanisms by which cigarette smoke is associated with these complications is relatively unknown.

• Oxygen increase after 48 hours of smoking cessation is supported by Davies, Latto & Jones (1984). The effects on the fetus after maternal cigarette smoking was stopped for 48 hours demonstrated that there was a subsequent reduction in carbooxyhaemoglobin and a decrease in haemoglobin oxygen affinity, which led to a significant increase of 8% in available oxygen over this period. These findings are a positive motivator to quit regardless of gestational age. Certainly health promotion techniques are more cost effective than supporting a baby in intensive care as a result of cigarette smoke negatively influencing its birth weight. It is reported that savings to the National Health Service (NHS) can amount to between three and six times the cost of providing smoking cessation support and counselling to the pregnant woman (Buck et al 1997).

Infants of families who smoke

Passive smoking almost certainly contributes to deaths from heart disease (Secretary of State 1998b). Asthma sufferers stand an increased risk of suffering an attack in smoky atmospheres and children, with no choice of inhalation, are particularly vulnerable. Infants of mothers who smoke run a twofold risk of developing asthma. Prenatal exposure is probably a greater influence on the development of asthma in later life (Cook, Strachan & Anderson 1997–1998). The Royal College of Physicians has estimated that approximately 17 000 hospital admissions per year of children under 5 years old are due to their parents' smoking behaviour (Secretary of State for Health 1998b). The incidence of sudden infant death syndrome is increased in infants exposed to passive smoke (Floyd et al 1991). As cigarette smoke passes freely into breast milk the breast-fed infant is exposed to its harmful effects (Lambers & Clark 1996).

Why is it advisable to stop smoking rather than cut down?

Many pregnant women believe that trying to change from a middle tar to a low tar brand of cigarette will cause less harm to themselves and their unborn baby (Maclaine & Macleod-Clark 1991). Although low tar yield produces low nicotine yield, this is not true of the more harmful chemical carbon monoxide. It is a fallacy to assume that low tar brands are safer. This may offer a false sense of security to smokers who may alter their smoking behaviour, number of cigarettes smoked, method of puffing and depth of inhalation to maintain the desired level of nicotine intake. An alternative perspective is offered by Li (1993), who proposes that fetal effects of cigarette smoke are dose related; therefore those who manage to cut down successfully should be praised. Trevett (1997), however, challenges the benefits of cutting down and suggests that outright cessation should be advised.

What midwives can do to help pregnant women change their smoking behaviour

Smoking continues to be a habit that is extremely difficult to change, despite increasing social pressure to do so. Models which look for consistency within individuals do not adequately account for the high rate of relapse following smoking cessation. The model of attitudinal and behavioural change adapted from the Prochaska & DiClemente model of change (1993) by the HEA (1994) can be used to enable the practitioner and woman to focus quickly and efficiently on an identified smoking behaviour stage (see Fig. 6.1).

As previously discussed in Chapter 3, this model identifies a number of stages that a person can go through when trying to change their behaviour. It also recognises that, for some people, change may involve cycling through these stages more than once (see Fig. 6.1). Women are more likely

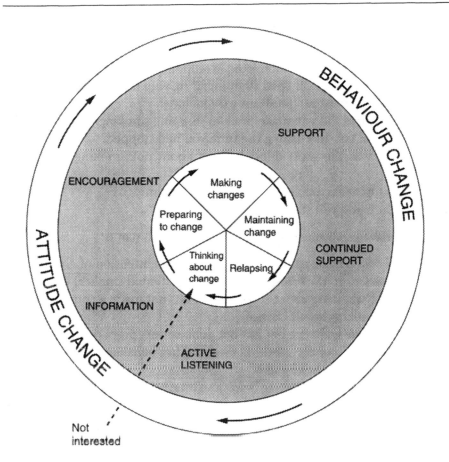

Figure 6.1
A model of attitude and behavioural change (from HEA 1994, after Prochaska & DiClemente 1986, with permission of the HEA)

to give up smoking in early rather than late pregnancy. They are more receptive at these times, either because of the initial enhanced desire to do what is best for their baby, or because of a readiness to use the opportunity when the appeal of smoking lessens owing to nausea (Mcknight & Merrett 1986). If preconception care is not available, midwives must utilise the booking visit to begin smoking cessation advice and counselling.

How do you begin?

In order to adopt the right approach it is important to assess the woman's readiness to change her smoking behaviour (see Fig. 6.1). This may consist of strategies which seek to elicit information from the client, encouraging the revelation of thoughts and feelings about smoking and giving up.

- Establish the nature of the woman's smoking behaviour.
- Establish the number of cigarettes smoked per day.
- Explore reasons for smoking. This may be followed by highlighting the dangers of cigarette smoke on the fetus. You may choose to begin your

sentence with: 'Although you have stated that you enjoy smoking are you aware that...'.
- Ask the woman if she is interested in stopping.
- Find out if she has ever tried stopping; if so, why didn't she succeed?
- Explore these reasons; questions may include:
  — What plans did you make prior to stopping smoking?
  — How did you feel during the time you had stopped?
  — What was the most difficult thing about not smoking during this time?
  — What benefits did you notice during this time?
  — What made you start smoking again?

You may have established at this point that the woman is:

1. not interested in stopping smoking and has no intention of changing her behaviour in the foreseeable future (contented smoker)
2. is seriously thinking about stopping but has not made a commitment to stop (thinking about change)
3. ready to make a change but has not done so yet (preparing to change)
4. ready to make a change and has modified her behaviour
5. or is maintaining the changes
6. or has resumed her smoking behaviour, maybe only after a brief moment of cessation.

Some women, regardless of which stage they are at in this behavioural change cycle, may inform the midwife that they have cut down since becoming pregnant or changed to a low tar brand. They may therefore feel that they have helped the situation by reducing their cigarette consumption. Although acknowledgement should be offered, such misconceptions should be challenged (see earlier section on cutting down).

You may now be in a position to identify the woman's position on the behavioural change cycle (identified by numbers 1–6 above). Consider the case studies in Boxes 6.1 and 6.2.

Reflection points

- Where is Janice on the behavioural change cycle?
- What issues would you need to discuss with her?
- How could you help her?

Box 6.1 **Case study: Janice**

Janice is 14 weeks' pregnant and smokes 20 cigarettes per day. She enjoys smoking, understands the risks involved and knows that at this moment in time she needs her cigarettes to reduce the stresses felt from being pregnant. She is concerned about her baby and would like to do everything she possibly can to give her baby the best start. Her partner and mother smoke and so does her sister, who had an 8 lb healthy baby girl after smoking throughout her pregnancy. She seeks reassurance that everything will be okay if she continues to smoke as she has already cut down.

Box 6.2 **Case study: Neice**

> Neice books for maternity care at 34 weeks' gestation; she smokes 15 cigarettes per day because she has a demanding home life. She has stopped on several occasions before, but there is always a crisis and the only way she copes is to start smoking again. To give up seems impossible; she asks for help but feels that it doesn't really matter about giving up now because she only has a few more weeks left before she has the baby.

Reflection points

- Where is Neice on the behavioural change cycle?
- What issues would you need to discuss with her?
- How could you help her?

Behavioural change strategies

Different strategies will be appropriate, depending on the woman's position in the cycle of behavioural change. The following is a guide.

Those identified as being contented smokers (1)

- Provide the woman with relevant and accurate information, advising and challenging misinformation, followed by further exploration of thoughts and feelings. This may reveal that the woman is not interested in changing her behaviour despite attempts to cut down during pregnancy.
- Women who are not interested in stopping smoking during pregnancy should have their decision respected. The midwife should not seek to impose guilt feelings.
- Damage limitation advice should be offered. The woman should be supported in developing strategies to reduce damage to other children and significant others who are exposed to sidestream smoke. Efforts should be channelled toward reducing the exposure of cigarette smoke to the baby once delivered.
- Inform the woman that she will be asked again about her smoking behaviour.
- Maintain appropriate records.

Those identified as thinking about change (2)

Women who are interested in stopping smoking should be provided with the help and support to progress toward changing their behaviour. The aim of the intervention skills here would be to help the woman progress to the next stage. This stage is a thinking stage; it may be useful to explore barriers which prevent progression toward cessation.

- Discuss the reasons why the woman smokes.
- Explore reasons for smoking cessation.
- Explore previous experiences of stopping and discuss positive and negative aspects of the planning stages.
- Explore strategies which will enhance the chances of stopping and staying stopped.

- Make the necessary changes to ensure stopping will be successful.
- Assess the situation with the woman; for example, how does it feel to have made the changes which may have involved informing family and friends of the proposed future change?
- Encourage the woman to decide on a stop date, encourage her to stick to it.
- Visual aids and self-help manuals include encouraging the woman to list all the positive and negative aspects about smoking, including the benefits to herself, her baby and significant others.
- Maintain appropriate records.

Offer continued support throughout the pregnancy. Offer the Quit Line number, which is a free service to callers within England which may offer additional support.

Those identified as preparing to change and making changes (3, 4)

Women who are in the preparation stage need specific help to stop smoking. This stage involves putting the planning into operation.

- Explore previous experiences of stopping and discuss positive and negative aspects of the planning stages.
- Make the necessary changes, this may include:
    — telling friends and family who can offer support
    — disposing of all the ashtrays, lighters and cigarettes in the house
    — recognising the cues for lighting up a cigarette, for example answering the telephone, having a cup of coffee, first thing in the morning, after an evening meal or when friends come to visit. Replace these triggers with something that is appealing and distractional; this must be left to personal preference.
- Plan a different daily routine to avoid smoking temptation areas.
- Explore strategies which will enhance the chances of stopping and staying stopped.
- Set the stop date and stick to it.
- Offer continued support throughout the remainder of the pregnancy.
- Offer the Quit Line number for additional support.
- Offer self-help manuals and visual aids which may provide additional support. (See Helping pregnant smokers quit: training for health professionals (HEA 1994).)
- Measure carbon monoxide levels in exhaled air (if a machine is available).
- Maintain appropriate records.

NB Plans which are extreme, like not mixing with friends because they smoke, may be unrealistic. Smoking may be an integral part of the woman's social life. It may be more productive and supportive, for example, if friends remained as a form of social support, but smoked outside the home or chose to socialise in venues that held both smoking and non-smoking areas.

Maintaining changes (5)

This stage involves encouraging and supporting the woman to maintain the change and may involve the use of some of the strategies utilised in the 'preparing to change and make changes' section (see above).

- In addition the woman would need to be assured of continued support.
- Encouragement needs to be given for maintaining the change.
- Reflection should take place on the positive aspects of not smoking – benefits and rewards.
- During 'danger' times when a cigarette was most enjoyed, encourage the woman to revisit the plan made when preparing to change and stick to it. This may include keeping busy or partaking in an activity. Eating less high fat foods, eating small amounts regularly and keeping active will help reduce the risk of excessive weight gain, which is sometimes experienced when food is substituted for cigarettes.

Resuming smoking behaviour (6)

If a woman has managed to stop smoking during pregnancy it is not uncommon for her to begin smoking again after the baby is born. The pressures of looking after a new baby, adjusting to motherhood and reduced social support are factors which predispose to resumption of smoking behaviour (Dunkley 1997). Midwives and health visitors should:

- encourage the woman to view her situation as a learning experience as opposed to an experience of failure: support and praise the length of time the woman remained a non-smoker, explore benefits and rewards, and discuss difficult moments and factors which caused her to resume her smoking behaviour
- assess the woman's readiness to change
- return to section on 'preparing to change' if appropriate.

The role of partner of the woman who smokes

The involvement of family members in counselling is vital. Partners in particular have a significant effect on the woman's motivation to change her smoking behaviour. Women find it extremely difficult to stop smoking during pregnancy if they have partners who smoke. Twenty per cent of women who smoked during pregnancy felt that they continued to smoke because their partners negatively influenced their ability to quit (Dunkley 1997). Women who are encouraged by their partners to stop smoking are more likely to succeed than women who are not supported. Since partners have such a significant effect on women's motivation to change their smoking behaviour, they should be involved in smoking cessation counselling if both the woman and the partner are willing. Partners can also be informed of the dangers of sidestream smoke, if they themselves smoke or continue to smoke. They may decide to stop smoking by way of support and encouragement and if so should be given the support and counselling necessary to make that change.

Misconceptions about smoking

Misconceptions which should be challenged include the following.

* **If you smoke you have smaller babies which are easier to deliver and short labours.** This is a common belief. Woman are more likely to have babies that are at risk of being sick and small. The length of labour is not determined by the size of the baby.
* **My mother smoked 20 cigarettes a day throughout all three of her pregnancies and they were all 8 pounds and over.** The placenta is a remarkable organ which has the ability to adjust its growth in order to compensate for the needs of the fetus in some women. Smoking results in hypoxia and to protect the fetus compensatory hypertrophy occurs. In order to maximise oxygen transfer, the surface area and vascularity increase and the diffusing distance of the placenta reduces.
* **Of course it's safe to breast feed when you smoke; smoke goes into your lungs and your bloodstream not into your breast milk.** Traces of nicotine have been found in breast milk in proportion to the number of cigarettes smoked. This can cause the infant to experience nausea and vomiting, and irritability. Failure to thrive may result owing to nicotine causing a suppression in lactation (Merenstein & Gardner 1998).
* **My husband says it's okay if he smokes around me because the air is generally slightly polluted anyway.** The air may be marginally polluted but the concentrations of carbon monoxide and nicotine are approximately 2.5-fold higher in sidestream smoke than in mainstream smoke. The fetus is at risk from passive exposure and therefore at an increased risk of intrauterine growth retardation.
* **I've cut down from smoking 20 a day to 15 cigarettes per day and I have changed to a low tar brand so my baby will be okay.** This is definitely not guaranteed. Low tar may mean low nicotine but carbon monoxide remains the same. To achieve the desired level of nicotine intake, smokers may alter their smoking behaviour – that is, the method of puffing and depth of inhalation.
* **I've only got a month to go before I have the baby; I feel bad because the baby is very small and they still want me to give up smoking. What's**

the point now the damage is already done? Stopping smoking even for 48 hours leads to a significant increase of 8% of available oxygen to the fetus.

A word of caution

You may find that it is difficult to establish where the woman is on the behavioural change cycle, as establishing this information requires two-way communication, trust, genuineness and empathy. An individualised approach to counselling about smoking cessation is the better approach. Exploration of thoughts and feelings is extremely important if the woman is to move forward toward a behavioural change. Remember that Rome was not built in a day! Women who are contented smokers will have increased awareness and damage limitation strategies to begin with. Those who are thinking about change may wish to give up but feel that, due to outside stressors and social deprivation, stopping what they consider to be their only enjoyment may be extremely difficult and they may require an abundance of help. Those who are preparing to change and those who are making changes should have explored strategies for staying stopped and need support and encouragement for maintenance. Ultimately the decision to modify the smoking behaviour must be that of the client. The midwife is purely a facilitator within that role.

Summary

- Twenty-four per cent of women smoke during pregnancy and only 33% give up whilst pregnant.
- Very few women give up smoking later on in the pregnancy.
- Pregnancy is considered an ideal time to help women who wish to give up smoking to do so successfully.
- Pregnancy is a good motivator to help women stop smoking.
- The government proposes that tackling smoking is central to improving health in Britain and has pledged funding of approximately £60 million toward delivering expert help to those most in need. Education and resource allocation will enable midwives to possess the confidence and skills necessary to interact effectively with women and their partners.
- Resources, time and commitment should be available for the service provision and there should be support from peers, superiors and professional bodies.
- Women find it extremely difficult to stop smoking during pregnancy if they have partners who smoke.
- Pregnant women have a high rate of encounters with the health care system. This continuous contact may offer an opportunity for smoking cessation. In order for such an intervention to be successful, however,

it should be relevant to the needs of the woman and based on an understanding of why women smoke during pregnancy.

- It is evident that there are many studies which have attempted to understand why pregnant women smoke and why they continue to smoke. Cigarette smoking among women is not so much an addiction but a way of life. Women may be more likely to use cigarettes during socialising to feel more confident.
- The dangers of passive smoking are quite profound and almost certainly contribute to deaths from heart disease.
- Smoking cessation intervention counselling during pregnancy may have a major impact on the female smoking prevalence, and consequently on the health of women and their offspring.
- Asthma sufferers stand an increased risk of suffering an attack in smoky atmospheres and children, with no choice over inhalation, are particularly vulnerable.
- Health professionals need to understand the process of behavioural change to facilitate the change process.
- Damage limitation should be high on the agenda of health professionals when engaged in smoking cessation counselling.
- Health education strategies used to help people stop smoking involving television programmes or leaflets have been found to be less effective than individual counselling techniques.
- In pregnancy the usual care providers, especially physicians and midwives, are well placed to provide smoking cessation interventions because of their regular contact with pregnant women.
- Health professionals greatly influence the decision of the woman to stop smoking.

References

Aaronson L, Mural C, Pfoutz S 1988 Seeking information where do pregnant women go? Health Education Quarterly 15:335–345

American College of Obstetrics and Gynecologists (ACOG) 1993 Smoking and reproductive health. ACOG technical bulletin no 180

Andres R 1996 The association of cigarette smoking with placenta praevia and abruptio placenta. Seminars in Perinatology 20(2):154–159

Arborelius E, Krakau I, Bremberg S 1992 Key factors in health counselling in the consultation. Family Practice 9(4):489–493

Backe B 1993 Maternal smoking and age. Effect on birth weight and risk for small for gestational age births. Acta Obstetrica Gynaecologia (Scand) 72:172–176

Benowitz N 1991 Nicotine replacement therapy during pregnancy. Journal of the American Medical Association 266(22):3174–3177

Blackburn S, Loper D 1992 Maternal fetal and neonatal physiology: a clinical perspective. W B Saunders, Philadelphia

Buck D, Godfrey C, Parrott S, Raw M 1997 Cost effectiveness of smoking cessation interventions. York & London, Centre for Health Economics, Health Education Authority, London

Callum C 1998 The United Kingdom smoking epidemic: deaths in 1995. Health Education Authority, London

Chapman S, Egger G 1993 Myth in cigarette advertising and health promotion. American Journal of Public Health 92(4):68–74

Cook D G, Strachan D P, Anderson R 1998 Health effects of passive smoking (Series of papers). Thorax (eds Britton J, Weiss S).

Davies J M, Latto P, Jones G 1984 Effects of stopping smoking for forty eight hours. British Medical Journal 2:355–356

Diamond A, Goddard E 1995 Smoking among secondary school children in 1994. HMSO, London

Dunkley J 1997 Training midwives to help pregnant women stop smoking. Nursing Times 93(5):64–66

Fiore M C, Bailey W C, Cohen S J et al 1996 Smoking cessation clinical practice guideline no 18, publication no 96–0692. Rockville MD, Agency for Health Care Policy and Research, US Department of Health and Human Services

Flay B, McFall S, Burton D, Cook T, Warnecke J 1993 Health behaviour changes through television: the roles of de facto and motivated selection processes. Journal of Health and Social Behaviour 34:322–335

Floyd R L, Zahniser S C, Gunter E P, Kendrick J S 1991 Smoking during pregnancy: prevalence, effects, and intervention strategies. Birth 18(1):48–53

Foster K, Lader D, Cheesbrough S 1997 Infant feeding 1995: Office for National Statistics. The Stationery Office, London

Fried P 1993 Pre-natal exposure to tobacco and marijuana: effects during pregnancy, infancy and early childhood. Clinical Obstetrics and Gynaecology 36(2):319–337

Gordon I 1997 Stopping them starting: evaluation of a community based project to discourage teenage smoking in Cardiff. Health Education Journal 56:42–50

Graham H 1993 When life's a drag – women, smoking and disadvantage. HMSO, London

Graham H, Hunt K 1998 Socio-economic influences on women's smoking status in adulthood: insights from the West of Scotland twenty-07 study. Health Bulletin 56:757–765

Greaves L 1996 Smokescreen – women's smoking and social control. Scarlet Press, London

Hackshaw A K, Law M, Wald N J 1997 The accummulated evidence on lung cancer and environmental tobacco smoke. British Medical Journal 315:980–988

Haglund B, Cnattinguis S 1990 Cigarette smoking as a risk factor for sudden infant death syndrome: a population based study. American Journal of Public Health 80:29–32

Health Education Authority (HEA) 1994 Helping pregnant smokers quit: training for health professionals. HEA, London

Health Education Authority (HEA) 1999 Smoking cessation guidelines for health professionals. HEA, London

Hecht S S, Carmella S G, Chen M L et al 1998 Metabolites of the tobacco-specific lung carcinogen abstracts papers. American Chemical Society 216:32

Lambers D, Clark K 1996 The maternal and fetal physiological effects of nicotine. Seminars in Perinatology 20(2):115–126

Li C 1993 The impact on infant birthweight and gestational age of continue-validated smoking reduction during pregnancy. Journal of the American Medical Association 269:1519–1524

Maclaine K, Macleod-Clark J 1991 Women's reason for smoking in pregnancy. Nursing Times 87(22) (May 29):39–42

Mcknight A, Merrett J D 1986 Smoking in pregnancy. A health education problem. Journal of Royal College of General Practitioners 36:161–164

Marsh A, Mackay S 1994 Poor smokers. Report no. 771. Policy Studies Institute, London

Mathai M, Vijayasri R, Babu S, Jeyaseelan L 1992 Passive maternal smoking and birth weight in a south Indian population. British Journal of Obstetrics and Gynaecology 99:182–184

Merenstein G B, Gardner S L 1998 Handbook of neonatal intensive care. Mosby, New York

Owen L, Scott P 1995 Barriers to good practice in smoking cessation work among pregnant women. Journal of the Institute of Health Education 33:110–112

Peacock J, Bland J, Anderson H 1991 Effects on birth weight of alcohol and caffeine consumption in smoking women. Journal of Epidemiology and Community Health 45(159):15–20

Poswillo D 1998 Report of the Scientific Committee on Tobacco and Health. The Stationery Office, London

Prochaska J, DiClemente C, Norcross C 1993 In search of how people change: applications to addictive behaviours. Addictions Nursing Network 5(1):3–16

Rush D, Ormet J, King J, Eiser J, Butler N 1992 A trial of health education aimed to reduce cigarette smoking among pregnant women. Paediatric and Perinatal Epidemiology 6:285–297

Secretary of State for Health 1998a Our healthier nation, a contract for health. A consultation. The Stationery Office, London

Secretary of State for Health 1998b Smoking kills. White paper. The Stationery Office, London

Silagy C, Lancaster T, Fowler G, Spiers I 1998a Effectiveness of training health professionals to provide smoking cessation interventions. Cochrane Review. In: The Cochrane Library issue 2 (updated quarterly). Oxford, Update Software

Silagy C, Mant D, Fowler G, Lancaster T 1998b Nicotine replacement therapy for smoking cessation. Cochrane review. In: The Cochrane Library issue 2 (updated quarterly). Oxford, Update Software

Svanberg B 1992 Smoking during pregnancy possibilities of prevention in antenatal care. International Journal of Technology Assessment in Health Care 8(1):96–100

Trevett N (ed) 1997 Smoking and pregnancy, a growing problem. Health Education Authority, London

University of York NHS Centre for Reviews and Dissemination 1998 Effectiveness Matters 3(1):13–14

Walsh R, Redman S 1993 Smoking cessation in pregnancy: do effective programmes exist? Health Promotion International 8(2):111–127

Wilms D, Best A 1991 Patient's perspectives of a physician delivered smoking cessation intervention. American Journal of Preventative Medicine 7:95–100

Recommended reading

Bolling K, Owen L 1997 Smoking and pregnancy. A survey of knowledge, attitudes and behaviour. Health Education Authority, London

Graham H 1998 Promoting health against inequality: using research to identify targets for intervention – a case study of women and smoking. Health Education Journal 57:292–302

This paper examines the socioeconomic differentials in women's smoking status through adolescence and across childhood. A policy framework for health promotion is identified which addresses issues related to female socioeconomic disadvantage.

Nicotinell 1993 Smoking mothers and young children: the hidden dilemma. Nicotinell, London

Prochaska J, DiClemente N 1994 Changing for the good. Morrow Publishing, Houston TX

This comprehensive guide to behaviour change offers the reader an opportunity to enhance current health-related behaviour change practices.

7 Alcohol use – safe measures during pregnancy?

Key themes

- Exploring ideas of safe levels of alcohol ingestion
- Effects of alcohol on the fetus; fetal alcohol syndrome
- Antenatal education; challenging misconceptions, the midwife's role
- Screening tests for alcohol misuse

Overview

This chapter will explore health issues in relation to alcohol ingestion during pregnancy and the teratogenic effects on the fetus. Health promotion strategies and the role of the midwife in helping women and their partners to make healthy lifestyle choices will also be explored in light of current evidence-based research. The reader will be encouraged to think critically about current advice, screening and guidance offered to women who drink alcohol during pregnancy. The value of using appropriate screening tools for alcohol misuse concludes the chapter. Prior knowledge of the following areas will enable the reader to understand the issues discussed in this chapter:

- how alcohol affects the functioning of the body
- the physiology of fetal development
- an appreciation of placental development and function.

Alcohol use during pregnancy

Drinking alcohol in Western communities forms part of a socially accepted pastime, sometimes to the extent of forced social exclusion if the behaviour is not shared. Over the past 20 years there has been an increasing trend towards higher levels of alcohol misuse in women within the United Kingdom. Pregnancy is often viewed as a time for lifestyle change and has been shown to motivate women to change their drinking behaviour in order to protect their unborn baby. The Royal College of Obstetricians and Gynaecologists (RCOG 1999) states that 90% of the population consume alcohol; during pregnancy this is reduced to 40–60%.

Midwives are ideally placed to help women make informed choices about drinking or abstaining from drinking alcohol during pregnancy. Recommendations from the RCOG (1999) provide guidance for midwives when offering advice and counselling to pregnant women about safe levels of alcohol use. However, there is no universal agreement of what constitutes a safe measure of alcohol during pregnancy. In light of the midwife's role, the provision of health promotion advice is therefore challenging when recommending safe alcohol measures. Heavy drinking during pregnancy is relatively rare in the United Kingdom (Abel & Sokol 1991). By way of contrast 7–15% of childbearing women in America are heavy drinkers, consuming on average 45 drinks per month (Jannke 1994). The identification of high risk groups (women who drink alcohol above levels which cause fetal alcohol-related effects) and the support needed fall within the remit of the midwife's role. Unfortunately, traditional screening is limited to establishing the drinking status and does not control for underestimation. The stigma attached to drinking during pregnancy may influence the accuracy of reporting drinking behaviour (Bruce, Adams & Shulman 1993). Identification of alcohol misuse is therefore unlikely.

Drinking alcohol during pregnancy – is there a safe measure?

Safe levels of alcohol consumption during pregnancy remain controversial. RCOG (1999) states that moderate alcohol consumption is a socially accepted behaviour in Western culture, where over 90% of the population consume alcohol. Categorising light, moderate and heavy drinkers in relation to the number of units of alcohol they consume a week does not provide an accurate indicator of alcohol misuse nor account for individual lifestyle and weight differences. Instead measures of alcohol, which have significant correlation with adverse fetal effects, will be used as a guideline for safety for the purpose of this chapter.

Evidence suggests that social alcohol consumption (approximately 14 units per week), has a negative effect on intrauterine fetal growth (Jacobson, Jacobson & Sokol 1994). The effects of lower levels of drinking during pregnancy are not well established. Some studies observing long term effects of alcohol consumption on the child show that moderate drinking, defined as seven to 13 drinks per week, increases the risk of behavioural effects in infancy and childhood (Halmesmaki, Raivio & Ylikorkala 1987, Waterson & Murray-Lyon 1989, Mitchell et al 1999). Other authors present evidence that long term neurological development of the infant may be compromised due to an extended period of fetal alcohol exposure (Becker et al 1994, Day & Richardson 1991, Forrest, Cdu & Florey 1991). It is difficult to determine whether cognition and behavioural function have been affected as a result of prenatal exposure to alcohol, or as a result of the environmental effects of alcohol-abusing parents. The results of other studies have demonstrated no risk with this level of drinking. Florey et al (1992) presented research evidence which shows that women who drink less than 10 units per week during pregnancy do not cause any harm to the fetus, providing this amount is ingested over several days. Other research evidence presents similar findings (Bell & Lumley 1989, Walpole, Zubrick & Pontre 1990).

Inconsistent research findings with regards to the effects of alcohol on the fetus (see next section) have influenced the conclusion that there is no safe alcohol intake limit (Bruce, Adams & Shulman 1993). In the United States of America (USA), alcohol consumption during pregnancy is not recommended (US Surgeon General 1981). There is a high prevalence of alcohol misuse in the United States which raises the incidence of fetal alcohol syndrome (FAS) to such an extent that it is the third leading cause of birth defects in the country following Down's syndrome and spina bifida (Bratton 1995). The incidence of FAS in France and Sweden is 1.3 and 1.7 per 1000 live births respectively (RCOG 1999). In England the RCOG (1999) suggests that alcohol consumption during pregnancy is safe, if its use is restricted. It advises that pregnant women should be careful about the amount of alcohol consumed and limit consumption to one alcoholic measure per day (seven units per week; see Box 7.1). The recommendation is based on research studies which show no adverse effect on pregnancy outcome with a consumption of less than 15 units of alcohol per week, and includes work carried out by Mills et al (1984) and Florey et al (1992). Women who choose to follow this recommendation should be advised that consumption should be evenly spaced. Saving the drink allowance for one occasion should be discouraged due to the potential of causing harm to the fetus (see next section). These guidelines are valid until December 2002, after which time there will be a period of review and update.

Box 7.1 **Units of alcohol (RCOG 1996)**

1 unit of alcohol approximately equals 8 g of absolute alcohol, which is equivalent to:

- half pint of ordinary strength beer, lager, cider, quarter pint of strong beer or lager
- quarter pint of strong beer or lager
- one small glass of wine
- one single measure of spirits
- one small glass of sherry

Fetal effects

Since ancient times there has been concern about drinking alcohol during pregnancy, with reference made to the prohibition of alcohol during pregnancy by religious authorities. As early as 1725 the Royal College of Physicians alerted the House of Commons of their concern regarding alcohol consumption during pregnancy causing unhealthy children (Warren & Bast 1988).

Women who drink 14 units of alcohol per week are considered to be at risk of preterm labour (Jacobson, Jacobson & Sokol 1994). It is, however, more convincing to suggest that the factors associated with intrauterine growth retardation are more likely to influence preterm labour. Although the frequency and extent of alcohol effects on pregnancy outcomes are variable, there is little dispute over the effects of high levels (14 units and above per week) of maternal alcohol intake on the fetus. Teratogenic effects of alcohol on the fetus are largely determined by the quantity of alcohol consumed and the timing of exposure in relation to the gestational age of the fetus.

A study by Tranmer (1985) highlights the effects on the fetus when seven units of alcohol are consumed within a short period of time. Six women who were scheduled for pregnancy termination took part in the study. The fetal umbilical blood levels and amniotic fluid levels were assessed for alcohol, after maternal ingestion of the equivalent of 2 ounces (57 g) of 80 proof distilled spirit, presented as one drink (equivalent to approximately 7.1 units). The results showed that there were similar levels of alcohol in the maternal blood and fetal umbilical cord. Alcohol was also present in the amniotic fluid. The researcher hypothesised that the fetus would take twice as long as its mother to get rid of the alcohol owing to its immaturity of 17 weeks' gestation.

Maternal alcohol consumption throughout pregnancy amongst heavy drinkers has been associated with altered fetal brain development and intrauterine growth retardation, which are classified as alcohol-related birth defects. Alcohol interferes with amino acid transport across the placenta, causing disruption in embryonic organisation. This interruption is thought to result in chronic uterine hypoxia and contributes to intrauterine growth retardation. Alcohol is also associated with diminished deoxyribonucleic acid (DNA) synthesis, disruption of protein synthesis and impaired cellular growth and as such contributes to fetal malformations (Pietrantoni & Knupple 1991) (see Fetal alcohol syndrome (FAS) below). Women who drink at this level are at an increased risk of delivering preterm infants, infants who suffer from intrauterine growth retardation and infants with congenital malformations (Halmesmaki, Raivio & Ylikorkala 1987, Jacobson, Jacobson & Sokol 1994, Shen, Hannigan & Kapatos 1999). Unfortunately, neonates who have suffered growth retardation during uterine life due to alcohol are less likely to exhibit catch up growth during early childhood than neonates who suffered the effects of intrauterine growth retardation for reasons other than alcohol (Jacobson et al 1993).

Animal studies have demonstrated that high levels of alcohol consumption result in behavioural and central nervous system anomalies, intrauterine growth retardation and morphological consequences (Becker et al 1994, Day & Richardson 1991). Evidence suggests that women who consume 42 units of alcohol weekly (six units per day, or 3 ounces (85 g)), near the time of conception and during the first few weeks after conception, have a significantly increased risk of their infant having FAS (Bruce, Adams & Shulman 1993, Waterson & Murray-Lyon 1989). Many women at this stage do not know that they are pregnant, therefore routine antenatal advice given at the antenatal booking appointment on alcohol consumption is too late to avert some of the effects of alcohol exposure to the fetus as a result of heavy drinking. It has, however, been shown that alcohol consumption at any stage of pregnancy has a negative impact on fetal development (Coles et al 1985). Studies have demonstrated that if there is a reduction in the amount of alcohol consumed during the mid trimester of pregnancy, the growth and development of the fetus could be modified (Petrakis 1987, Smith et al 1987). Reynolds et al (1995) suggest that damage to the fetus can be minimised even if there is a reduction in the amount of alcohol consumed later in pregnancy. It is therefore useful to continue to reassure and counsel women about reducing or abstaining from alcohol consumption throughout pregnancy. This is of particular relevance to those who are alcohol dependent or those who have engaged in binge drinking during pregnancy, prior to confirmation.

Fetal alcohol syndrome

The most serious outcome of prenatal alcohol exposure is FAS. This is reported to occur only in infants of women who have chronic alcohol problems, defined as dependence or abuse, and continue this behaviour throughout pregnancy. As early as 1967 research studies identified that the offspring of alcoholic parents suffered from neurological dysfunction, mental retardation, behavioural disorders, facial anomalies and an increased risk of infant mortality (Warren & Bast 1988). It was only in 1973 that the symptoms and abnormalities were labelled as FAS. The manifestations of the syndrome vary depending on the amount of alcohol consumed. Queenan & Hobbins (1996) define fetal alcohol syndrome as the presence of at least one abnormality in each of three categories: growth retardation before and after birth, central nervous system abnormalities and midfacial hypoplasia.

In mild cases there are slight physical and neurological anomalies, which include reduced attention focusing, mild developmental delay and occasionally hyperactivity. In severe cases with large amounts of alcohol consumption (14 units and above per week), characteristic features are apparent. These include: abnormal facial features, microcephaly, epicanthal folds, short upturned nose, maxillary hypoplasia, elongated midface, micrognathia and a thin upper lip, cardiac septal defects, minor limb abnormalities such as nail dysplasia and a shortened fifth digit. Growth deficiencies are also apparent, both pre- and postnatally (indicated by measurements below the third percentile for gestational age). Neurological disorders present as severe mental retardation, seizures, hyperactivity and developmental delays (Bratton 1995). Not all affected children have visible facial abnormalities and, if they do, although detected at birth the abnormalities are more distinguishable between 8 months and 8 years of age (Streissguth 1992). As the children progress into adulthood the features become less pronounced. Unfortunately, neurological disorders and cognitive delays persist throughout life (Shen, Hannigan & Kapatos 1999, Chang et al 1998).

Immediate postnatal care of the neonate

Risk assessment strategies may identify at-risk cases, but all too often a history of alcohol abuse is difficult to obtain. Sometimes therefore, subtle signs of FAS may go undetected and could present as learning difficulties during school years.

The fetus that has been exposed to alcohol just before birth may show signs of withdrawal during the early neonatal period. Clinical signs include: low apgar score, tremors, jitteriness, irritability, seizures, increased respiratory rate, increased muscle tone, abnormal reflexes and decreased sucking abilities. Some infants have disturbed sleep patterns (Smith & Eckardt 1991). Large quantities of maternal alcohol consumption are associated with neonatal lethargy, drowsiness and affected motor development (Sokol & Martier 1996). Vigilant observation and screening in the early neonatal period may help to reduce further complications. Antenatal screening for 'risky drinking' behaviour may help to reduce differential diagnosis and/or clarify suspicious non-specific signs and symptoms (Box 7.2). Women who breast feed are advised to avoid feeding their babies within 1 to 2 hours of alcohol intake.

A need for appropriate education

Alcohol is often used as a coping strategy for the temporary relief of stressful life circumstances. Amounts of alcohol ingestion vary according to individual needs and desires. Use of alcohol is commonplace and forms part of Western social norms. The difference between acceptable drinking and problem drinking is difficult to define. Problem drinking may occur as a

Discussion questions

- How do you establish the drinking status of women antenatally?

- What issues do you include in your discussion when discussing safe measures of alcohol intake with antenatal women?

- How does the risk assessment tool you currently use to screen for 'risky drinking' behaviour compare with the screening tests discussed on page 140?

Box 7.2 **Case study: Oliver**

Oliver was delivered by caesarean section for fetal distress. Despite a low Apgar score he responded well to basic resuscitation and had no further problems.

Twenty-four hours postdelivery, Oliver's mother was concerned by his one unsuccessful attempt to feed since delivery and informed the midwife. The midwife noted through clinical observation that Oliver was jittery, lethargic, drowsy and difficult to rouse. She immediately suspected hypoglycaemia and proceeded to take a blood sugar test.

NB The drinking status of Oliver's mother was recorded in antenatal records as 'social drinker'. In actual fact what she did not disclose was that she consumed 21 units of alcohol per week.

result of moderate drinking patterns in some, whereas those who drink heavily may not be viewed as problem drinkers if they appear to function 'normally' within society. Socially accepted behaviour may include binge drinking and still be described by the individual as a moderate intake. Individual perceptions and ideas about alcohol consumption influence the nature of information given by clients when answering questions about alcohol use antenatally.

It is not unfair to infer that some people believe a glass of wine a day during pregnancy causes no harm to the fetus. Overwhelming evidence suggests that this level of alcohol consumption causes no immediate, adverse effects on the fetus (RCOG 1999), but inconsistencies in research evidence in relation to long term sequelae of alcoholic effects present an element of risk when consuming any levels of alcohol during pregnancy (Bruce, Adams & Shulman 1993). The woman's perception of what constitutes a safe measure is varied. Lelong et al (1995), in a study of 175 women, identified that 60% of women categorised as light drinkers thought that two alcoholic drinks per day constituted a reasonable level of consumption during pregnancy. This level of consumption is indicative of high risk drinking, consuming 14 units per week, which is associated with the mild effects of FAS (Bratton 1995).

Also, individual perceptions of a single measure of alcohol vary enormously. Invariably pub measures provide a more accurate interpretation of units of alcohol than home measures, which are usually poured freehand and not measured. Also the type of glass used at home has the potential to hold more alcohol than the single pub measure of one unit. Women may report drinking one glass of alcohol per day, but in actual fact consume three units in one poured measure. This was further supported by Lelong et al (1995) who asked 117 women how much wine and beer they felt it was safe to consume during pregnancy. Only 6% of women did not allow at least one drink per day. 11% of women felt that consuming three glasses of wine a day was reasonable and 17% of women felt the same about beer.

It was generally considered more acceptable to drink more beer than wine. Women who ordinarily drank higher quantities of alcohol were more likely to judge higher levels of consumption during pregnancy to be acceptable (Lelong et al 1995).

Another misconception is that the alcohol does not reach the fetus. Alcohol is a water soluble nervous system depressant that has no respect for the placental barrier and crosses it freely. As highlighted earlier, Tranmer (1985) detected alcohol in the fetal umbilical cord and amniotic fluid of the fetus. Another common misconception is that beer is not as potent as hard liquor (e.g. whisky, brandy, etc.), and therefore can be ingested freely during pregnancy (Brooten, Peters & Glatts 1987, Lelong et al 1995). Midwives must remind women that no type of alcohol is safer than any other. Challenging inaccurate ideas about alcohol consumption can help to correct misconceptions and provide an opportunity for education and counselling.

Health promotion in practice

It is well documented that a large proportion of women stop drinking or reduce their alcohol consumption during pregnancy (RCOG 1999). Approximately 20% of women will drink some alcohol during pregnancy, even though there is no identified universally accepted safe measure (Stratton, Howe & Battaglia 1996). Many women perceive alcohol to be a positive part of their social lives and as such it is unrealistic to expect them to stop drinking without providing appropriate education, advice and support. Heavy drinkers are more likely to book for maternity care late into their pregnancies and generally need intensive counselling and possibly referral to specialist agencies to help them reduce alcohol consumption during pregnancy (Russell et al 1994). Others, however, may choose not to book for maternity care. Health promotion strategies used to raise public awareness about the teratogenic effects of alcohol during pregnancy have demonstrated some success. A study comparing the impact of the Federal Alcohol Beverage Warning Label on multiparous and primiparous women in the USA, revealed that multiparous women who drink more than 14 units per week are less likely to change their drinking behaviour than primiparous women who drink the same amount, despite knowledge of the teratogenic effects of alcohol on the fetus. The researchers suggest that this is because multiparous women have delivered children whom they perceive to have suffered no ill effects of alcohol and therefore question the need to change their drinking behaviour during subsequent pregnancies (Hankin et al 1996). The findings not only support the ideas that behavioural change is influenced by previous experience but also that the provision of information alone does not cause behavioural change.

Screening, assessment and advice during pregnancy have been shown to be effective in reducing alcohol consumption (Handmaker, Miller & Manicke 1999). It is suggested that health professionals should identify and reach the small percentage of women who are heavy drinkers and help them to reduce their alcohol consumption during the periconception period. By far the biggest challenge, however, is helping heavy drinkers who conceive unplanned pregnancies. It could be argued that health promotion strategies should be targeted toward all women of childbearing age. The utilisation of family-planning clinics, general practitioner surgeries, school nurses, school curricula and widespread media publicity to target this group may enable a large proportion of the population to be aware of the adverse effects of binge drinking.

It is suggested that, because a safe limit of alcohol consumption during pregnancy has not been defined universally, a recommendation of abstinence is the only safe measure (Warren & Bast 1988 Bradley & Bennett 1997). Health campaigns to deliver this message could prove costly, however. The risk of the problem has therefore been analysed in relation to benefit and cost effectiveness in many areas. A study carried out in Bristol, England, on alcohol during pregnancy (James et al 1995) reported that, out of a population of 500 women, the majority (92%), consumed less than 10 grams per day (approximately 1.25 units). The most any mother consumed was 18 grams per day (just below two units). There was no association between the low level of alcohol consumption and adverse pregnancy outcomes. There was also no association between alcohol consumption and smoking. The researchers concluded that there was little evidence to support the finances involved in delivering a health education campaign to all women in Bristol. Concerted efforts were directed only toward moderate to heavy drinkers, with proven risks (James et al 1995). Jacobson et al (1993) presented a strong argument for all women of childbearing age to be screened for alcohol consumption when they present for any form of health care, regardless of their reproductive status. This involved questions about alcohol use incorporated into initial history interviews. This approach would undoubtedly reach large members of the population and serve as a form of risk management and promotion of healthy lifestyles.

General practitioners have extensive access to the general population and as such are ideally placed to screen patients for alcohol misuse and raise awareness about the consequences of binge drinking (Deehan, Marshall & Strang 1998). Wider availability and accessibility of preconception care, however, would enable the midwife to advise and support women. Brief interventions in a primary care setting including preconception care, has been shown to be as effective in promoting a healthy behavioural change, in comparison to more extensive treatment for alcohol problems (Miller & Rollnick 1991). The midwife should provide current appropriate advice to all clients on alcohol use during pregnancy regardless of the suggested categories of light, moderate or heavy drinkers. Guided by numerous studies which present inconsistent findings, it would be fair to surmise that midwives should inform client groups that no universally safe level of drinking during pregnancy has been established. The guidance measures from the RCOG (1999), however, should be offered. If clients have already consumed large volumes of alcohol prior to the booking visit and have not had access to preconception care, the midwife should offer guidance, support and reassurance to the client and facilitate, through counselling, a non-alcoholic approach for the remainder of the pregnancy. Some clients who would still like to have the occasional alcoholic drink during pregnancy would have made an informed decision to do so.

Interventions

There is a general trend toward underestimation of alcohol consumption (Ernhart et al 1988, Stoler & Holmes 1999). This underestimation and underreporting will inhibit the identification of high risk drinkers. Utilisation of a screening tool such as the T-ACE questionnaire (see Screening tests, p. 141) has been found to identify correctly 70% of heavy drinkers during pregnancy and as such can be considered a useful screening tool (RCOG 1999). The value of brief interventions should not be underestimated; they have been found to be cost effective in targeting the most excessive drinkers (Deehan, Marshall & Strang 1998).

Intervention programmes designed to reduce alcohol consumption amongst pregnant women have generally involved public information campaigns. Whilst reaching large numbers of the community, substantial behavioural change may not be achieved. Effective screening programmes which identify light, moderate and heavy drinkers would enable the appropriate counselling strategies to be used for each identified group. Prenatal intervention programmes, including education and counselling and group therapy, have indicated that 67–76% of participants including high risk drinkers reduce or abstain from alcohol consumption (Smith & Coles 1991). Intervention techniques consisting of a nine-step self help manual and a 10 minute education session, influenced a higher alcohol quit rate, of 88%. (Usual support methods presented a quit rate of 60%.) The intervention, however, was more effective amongst those categorised as light drinkers (Reynolds et al 1995). Research studies have highlighted that the most significant people to help decrease alcohol consumption are: the midwife, general practitioner and the woman's husband. Most women recognise that alcohol could be harmful to the fetus but heavy drinkers are less likely than light drinkers to cite the effects of alcohol on the fetus (Lelong et al 1995, Deehan, Marshall & Strang 1998). Prevention programmes can only be appropriately tailored to reach and effectively modify behaviour of high risk groups if information on demographic details, social structure and psychosocial characteristics associated with drinking are taken into account. To influence the reduction or cessation of a potential coping strategy has moral implications. The health promotion approach should consider socioeconomical factors and explore appropriate replacement coping strategies. Heavy drinkers should be encouraged to cut down their alcohol consumption and discouraged from drinking to the point of intoxication. Hankin & Sokol (1995) state that the teratogenic effects of alcohol are dose related and drinking that poses the greatest concern is drinking which raises the blood alcohol levels high enough and for long enough to produce fetal damage. The precise level of blood alcohol varies with each individual; therefore difficulty arises when determining precisely which levels produce fetal damage.

In order to afford the best strategies for alcohol cessation during pregnancy, specifically for those who are moderate to heavy drinkers, it is essential that a clear understanding is achieved about the various behavioural components of maternal drinking and the influences surrounding them. Influencing factors have been identified and include the following (adapted from May 1995).

• Women who have partners who drink heavily are encouraged to do so themselves (Lelong et al 1995, Wilsnack et al 1991).
• Women who are of low socioeconomic status have been found to have the highest rates of infants with FAS (Bingol et al 1987, Sokol, Martier & Ager 1989).
• Occupational norms of drinking and unemployment generally consist of occupations that are male dominated and encourage heavy drinking among females (Wilsnack & Wilsnack 1992, Wilsnack et al 1991).
• Polysubstance misuse and cigarette use are commonly associated with heavy alcohol users (Day, Cottreau & Richardson 1993, Godel et al 1992).
• Cultural patterns of alcohol consumption are highlighted by the finding that cultures which tolerate heavy drinking have high rates of FAS (May et al 1983).

It is suggested that efforts to stop heavy alcohol consumption during pregnancy have been predominantly clinic based and do not consider the wider socioeconomic influences and the importance of the overall life cycle of the drinking female. Being aware of the context in which women drink and the patterns of drinking may positively influence the intervention strategy.

A multilevel, comprehensive prevention programme with primary, secondary and tertiary prevention components sought to reduce FAS and/or fetal alcohol-related birth defects (ARBD) (May 1995). Specific goals of this programme were to provide reinforcement strategies and controls,

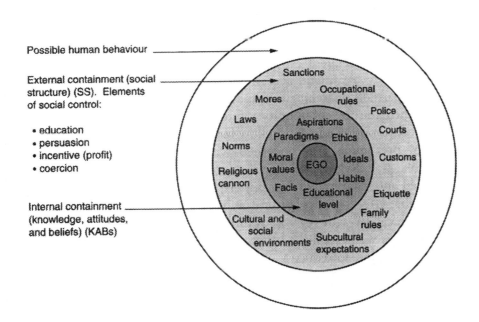

Possible human behaviour

External containment (social
structure) (SS). Elements
of social control:

- education
- persuasion
- incentive (profit)
- coercion

Internal containment
(knowledge, attitudes,
and beliefs) (KABs)

Sanctions
Occupational rules
Mores
Police
Laws
Aspirations
Courts
Paradigms   Ethics
Norms
Moral   Ideals   Customs
values   EGO
Religious   Habits
cannon
Facis   Educational   Etiquette
level
Cultural and   Family
social   rules
environments   Subcultural
expectations

Figure 7.1
**Levels of influence
and control over an
individual's behaviour
relevant to FAS and
ARBD prevention
(concepts adapted
from Reckless 1967,
with permission of
Appleton Century
Crofts)**

which overlap to prevent ARBD. The purposes of this programme were to
view the influences of alcohol use from an holistic viewpoint, ranging from
the woman's identity, innermost thoughts and her drive, which were
considered to be central (see Fig. 7.1). This is confounded by a surrounding
circle called the 'internal containment complex', which is made up of existing
knowledge, attitudes and beliefs about drinking, which serves to guide and
channel an individual's thoughts. This is further confounded by an outer
circle or third level referred to as the 'concept of external containment'.
The outer circle is made up of societal rules and family and cultural rules,
which also provide definitions of how to behave in certain situations.
Internal and external containment are thought to prevent an individual
from behaving in a way which would cause ARBD. Each level of prevention
is matched with a level of maternal drinking.

Primary levels are based on non-drinkers and light drinkers and as such
these methods can be applied to the general public. The intent is to reduce
the occurrences or incidence of the health problem. The strategies include:
public education, electronic and printed media to support primary health
care teams in schools, churches and civic groups, elimination of alcohol
advertising, particularly adverts linking and glamorising alcohol with sexual
behaviour, environmental changes which do not support heavy drinking
and promote socioeconomic improvement and other activities which
promote the value of human life and health. Secondary levels of prevention

are concerned with detecting the early onset of binge drinking or heavy drinking and promoting intervention strategies which will prevent problem drinking and subsequent ARBD. The strategies to prevent this would include: quality treatment, accessibility for the special needs of women and their partners, matching clients to treatments based on the level and type of their misuse, community reinforcement approach, monitoring of alcohol consumption and counselling for pregnant heavy drinkers. Tertiary levels of prevention are concerned with the worst possible situation already existing. Referral to specialist agencies would be necessary with: continued antenatal midwifery support, education and counselling about the possible effects of alcohol on the baby, support and care postnatally, further education with regards to birth control and control of the drink problem. It is well established that those women who are heavy drinkers are the least likely to reduce their alcohol consumption (Day, Cottreau & Richardson 1993, Serdula et al 1991). This situation is more apparent in the USA where the prevalence of FAS remains high. Prevention strategies cannot hope to succeed unless they include the appropriate services for other drug use including cigarette smoking. Studies have highlighted that alcohol use during pregnancy is closely associated with smoking and illicit drug use (Forrest, Cdu & Florey 1991, National Institute on Drug Abuse 1994).

Punitive interventions

Preventative strategies based on punitive action gained momentum in the USA in the early 1990s. Women were arrested and prosecuted for manslaughter for prenatal child abuse due to heavy drinking during pregnancy (Blume 1996). Despite moral and ethical concerns the socioeconomic circumstances of many women who abuse alcohol during pregnancy are hard, and alcohol use is purely a coping strategy to continue with the hardships of their designated inadequate social positions. Punishment of this nature would only serve to fuel anger and stress and invoke further abuse to cope with provoked new emotions.

Screening

Screening should be an integral part of the booking interview or pre-conception care consultation. The aim of screening in this context would be to identify women who drink levels of alcohol that have been shown through research to be teratogenic to the fetus. Appropriate intervention strategies can then be utilised to promote short and long term gain. Unfortunately the accurate reporting of alcohol consumption during pregnancy is only as good as the professional seeking the information, the phrasing of the question and the midwife's attitude to alcohol intake which affects the woman's response to the question. Research has demonstrated that if questions about alcohol consumption are asked in a direct, non-judgemental way then women are more likely to answer honestly (Weiner, Morse & Garrido 1989). A maternal and infant health survey revealed that women who drink while they are pregnant are more likely to be white, educated, of a high income level, married and smokers (Centres for Disease Control and Prevention 1998). Health professionals involved in initiating questions in relation to alcohol ingestion should have a clear understanding about their own thoughts and ideas to enable a clear, unambiguous, non-judgemental approach.

Asking questions about alcohol consumption

Questions like 'You don't drink do you?' invite a closed, defensive response, which is likely to produce a negative answer. The client may feel intimidated, and conform to the perceived request of the health professional to say 'no'. Hungerford, Hymbaugh & Floyd (1994) suggest that defensive responses can be avoided by assuming that all women drink alcohol. This is thought to imply that the health professional considers it to be a socially accepted behaviour. Some cultural groups, however, may find this assumption offensive. This approach may therefore work for some, but cause offence to others.

A popular direct question which is unassuming may include, 'Do you drink alcohol?' The responses may include the following.

- 'I drink socially.'
- 'Just a few a week.'
- 'Not really.'
- 'A moderate amount.'
- 'A few glasses of wine.'

The responses do not provide very much information and are open to subjective interpretation. Advice and counselling may be inappropriate if exploration of meaning does not follow.

Screening tests

Screening tests are a useful method to assess alcohol levels which present as risk drinking. They are used to measure input and output levels of alcohol and provide a useful vehicle for identification of those who abuse and/or are dependent on alcohol. They help to separate those who are in need of further assessment from those who are not.

The TWEAK test seeks to identify risk drinking among women (Chan

Reflection points

- How do you define alcoholism?
- Is it a disease or a moral issue?
- What does a female alcoholic look like?
- How comfortable are you talking about alcohol consumption during pregnancy?
- What attitudes do you convey when you initiate the question?
- What do you do with the answers?

(From Uhrich 1997)

Box 7.3 **TWEAK test**

T Tolerance: How many drinks does it take before you begin to feel the first effects of the alcohol? (record number of drinks)
W Have your friends or relatives worried or complained about your drinking in the past year?
E Eye-opener: Do you sometimes take a drink in the morning when you first get up?
A Amnesia: Are there times when you drink and can't remember afterward what you said or did?
K(C) Do you sometimes feel the need to cut down on your drinking?

Appropriate uses
Designed for use with pregnant women. Appropriate as a screen for women who are abusive drinkers
Scoring
T—2 points if five or more drinks without passing out
W—2 points for yes
E, A and K(C)—1 point each for yes

Two or more out of a possible 7 is considered a positive indication of risk drinking for women

Administration
Can be self-administered. Brief. Simple to score

Cautions
May not identify women who are in the early stages of drinking problems. Does not collect information on the level of intake

(Reprinted by permission of the publisher from Chan et al 1993 Use of the TWEAK test in screening for alcoholism/heavy drinking in three populations. Alcoholism, Clinical and Experimental Research 17(6):1188–1192. Copyright 1993 by QUADRANT HEALTHCOM Inc.)

et al 1993) (Box 7.3); it can be used to detect outcome quickly and consists of five questions. The questions are very much focused on the results of drinking behaviour. Scores of two or more are indicative of risky behaviour. The T-ACE questionnaire, designed by Sokol, Martier & Ager (1989), is a similar screening test and consists of four questions, three of which are synonymous with the TWEAK test.

The T-ACE test assesses tolerance of alcohol, other people's opinions of the individual's drinking habits, the individual's thoughts about cutting down and the need for a drink first thing in the morning. Scores of two or more are indicative of risky behaviour. This questionnaire is advocated for use during pregnancy by the RCOG (1999). By assessing tolerance both questionnaires evade a questioning approach which may trigger denial or underestimation of alcohol intake. Self-administered questionnaires raise the problem of literacy skills, which may cause non-compliance with regards to completion. Midwives may choose to work through the brief tool with the woman, but research suggests that women are more likely to report alcohol-related behaviour accurately in self-administered questionnaires (Russell et al 1994).

A research study comparing the efficacy of the TWEAK and the T-ACE questionnaires in detecting risk drinking among pregnant women found relatively little difference between the two. The study, which included a population of 4743 pregnant women, validated both tools, but suggested that the TWEAK questionnaire may outperform the T-ACE with regards to sensitivity (Russell et al 1994).

Discussing the nature of alcohol use, patterns of drinking and the context in which alcohol is used would be helpful in working toward decrease or cessation of drinking behaviour. A screening tool should be utilised at each antenatal visit, not only to determine risk but to support progress made. Although this may prove time consuming, the benefits far outweigh the risks. Maternity provider units should critically consider adopting this method of screening as an integral part of health improvement. Finances and resources, however, often present stumbling blocks toward full integration, particularly when an acceptable level of drinking during pregnancy has been established in England. The postnatal visit can be used as a forum for continued support for the woman and her partner. If alcohol is used as a coping strategy to reduce the effects of stress then strategies aimed at reducing the stressors may be the first step in reducing alcohol consumption. For those identified as heavy drinkers, it may be appropriate to refer the woman to Alcoholics Anonymous for specialist help, but reassurance must be given of continued midwifery support to reduce any feelings of rejection.

Summary

- Appropriate screening strategies should form an integral part of the booking history or preconception consultation for all pregnant women, to exclude those whose alcohol intake poses a risk during pregnancy.
- Maternity provider units should critically consider adopting this method of screening as an integral part of health improvement.
- Finances and resources often present stumbling blocks toward full integration of screening for alcohol, particularly when an acceptable level of drinking during pregnancy has been established in England.

- Alcohol exposure during the first trimester of pregnancy ranging from two or more drinks a day to consuming six or more drinks a day will lead to mild to severe forms of FAS. Evidence relating to lower levels of alcohol consumption is inconsistent.
- Small amounts of alcohol, less than two alcoholic drinks per day, may cause neurological abnormalities.
- Because there is an element of risk involved when consuming even small amounts of alcohol women should be advised to stop drinking prior to conception and maintain this until after delivery.
- Brief interventions have the potential to reduce individual consumption, with subsequent public health benefits.
- Midwives are ideally placed to inform women of the potential hazards of alcohol consumption in pregnancy but an understanding that providing information does not translate to lifestyle change is important.
- The wider socioeconomic circumstances of each individual must be taken into account if support and counselling are to be effective.
- Very often pregnancy is a turning point for many women – a new life and new beginnings. The midwife can be proactive in helping women to make their choices in the preconception period or during the antenatal period about healthier lifestyles and encourage and support them in their attempts to change.
- Informing the woman of safe measures of alcohol can be difficult when research evidence presents inconsistencies. The RCOG guidelines suggest that ingesting one unit of alcohol a day is a safe level.
- Midwives should present information to women to enable them to make an informed choice about the level of alcohol they wish to consume within the safe limits advocated by the RCOG. Abstinence of alcohol during pregnancy, however, is the only true safe measure.

References

Abel E L, Sokol R J 1991 A revised conservative estimate of the incidence of fetal alcohol syndrome and its economic impact. Alcoholism, Clinical and Experimental Research 15:514–524

Becker H C, Randall C L, Salo A L et al 1994 Animal research; charting the course for fetal alcohol syndrome. Alcohol Health Research World 18(1):10–16

Bell R, Lumley J 1989 Alcohol consumption, cigarette smoking and fetal outcome in Victoria, 1989. Community Health Studies 13:484–491

Bingol N, Schuster C, Fuchs J et al 1987 Influence of socio-economic factors on the occurrence of fetal alcohol syndrome. Advances in Alcohol and Substance Abuse 6:105–118

Blume S 1996 Preventing fetal alcohol syndrome: where are we now? Addiction 91(4): 473–475

Bradley S, Bennett N 1997 Preparation for pregnancy: an essential guide. Argyll Publishing, Glendaruel

Bratton R L 1995 Fetal alcohol syndrome: how you can help prevent it. Postgraduate Medicine 98(5):197–200

Brooten D, Peters M A, Glatts M 1987 A survey of nutrition, caffeine, cigarette and alcohol intake in early pregnancy in an urban clinical population. Journal of Nurse Midwifery 32(2):85–90

Bruce F, Adams M M, Shulman H B 1993 Alcohol use before and during pregnancy. American Journal of Preventative Medicine 9(5):267–272

Centres for Disease Control and Prevention 1998 Sociodemographic and behavioural characteristics associated with alcohol consumption during pregnancy – United States. Morbidity and Mortality Weekly Report 44:261–265

Chan A W K, Pristach E A, Welte J W, Russell M 1993 Use of the TWEAK test in screening for alcoholism/heavy drinking in three populations. Alcoholism, Clinical and Experimental Research 17(6):1188–1192

Chang G, Wilkins-Haug L, Berman S, Goetz M, Behr H, Hiley A 1998 Alcohol use and pregnancy: improving identification. Obstetrics and Gynecology 91:892–898

Coles C, Smith I, Fernhoff P, Falek A 1985 Neonatal neurobehavioural characteristics as correlates of maternal alcohol use during gestation. Alcoholism, Clinical and Experimental Research 9:454–460

Day N L, Richardson G A 1991 Prenatal alcohol exposure: a continuum of effects. Seminars in Perinatology 15(4):271–279

Day N, Cottreau C, Richardson G 1993 The epidemiology of alcohol, marijuana and cocaine use among women of childbearing age and pregnant. Clinical Obstetrics and Gynaecology 36(2):232–245

Deehan A, Marshall J, Strang J 1998 Tackling alcohol misuse: opportunities and obstacles in primary care. British Journal of General Practice 48:1779–1782

Florey C, Taylor D, Bolumar F et al (eds) 1992 Euromac. A European concerted action: maternal alcohol consumption and its relation to the outcome of pregnancy and child development at 18 months. International Journal of Epidemiology 21(4) suppl 1:17–21

Forrest F, Cdu V, Florey D 1991 Reported social alcohol consumption during pregnancy and infant's development at 18 months. British Medical Journal 303(679): 22–26

Godel J, Pabst H, Hodges P, Johnson K, Froese G, Joffries M 1992 Alcohol in pregnancy. Canadian Medical Association Journal 147(2):181–188

Halmesmaki E, Raivio K, Ylikorkala O 1987 Patterns of alcohol consumption during pregnancy. Obstetrics and Gynecology 69:594–597

Handmaker N, Miller W, Manicke M 1999 Findings of a pilot study of motivational interviewing with pregnant drinkers. Journal of Studies on Alcohol 60(2):285–287

Hankin J, Sokol R 1995 Identification and care of problems associated with alcohol ingestion in pregnancy. Seminars in Perinatology 19(4):286–292

Hankin J, Firestone J, Sloan J et al 1996 Heeding the alcoholic beverage warning label during pregnancy: multiparae versus nulliparae. Journal of Studies on Alcohol (March):171–177

Hungerford D, Hymbaugh K, Floyd R 1994 Alcohol abuse during pregnancy. The Female Patient 19:27–50

Jacobson J, Jacobson S, Sokol R et al 1993 Teratogenic effects of alcohol on infant development. Alcoholism, Clinical and Experimental Research 7:174–183

Jacobson J L, Jacobson S W, Sokol R J 1994 Effects of prenatal exposure to alcohol, smoking and illicit drugs on postpartum somatic growth. Alcoholism, Clinical and Experimental Research 18:317–373

James D, Greenwood R, McCabe K, Mahomed K, Golding J 1995 Alcohol consumption during pregnancy in Bristol. Journal of Obstetrics and Gynaecology 15:84–87

Jannke S 1994 When the mother-to-be drinks. Childbirth Instructor Magazine 4(1):28–31

Lelong N, Kaminski M, Chwalow J, Bean K, Subtil D 1995 Attitudes and behaviour of pregnant women and health professionals towards alcohol and tobacco consumption. Patient Education and Counselling 25:39–49

May P 1995 A multiple-level, comprehensive approach to the prevention of fetal alcohol syndrome and other related birth defects. International Journal of the Addictions 30(12):1549–1602

May P, Hymbaugh K, Aase J, Samet J 1983 Epidemiology of fetal alcohol syndrome among American Indians of the Southwest. Social Biology 30:374–387

Miller W R, Rollnick S 1991 Motivational interviewing: preparing people to change addictive behaviour. Guilford Press, New York, pp 30–35

Mills J L, Graubard B I, Harley E E, Rhoads G G, Berendes H W 1984 Maternal alcohol consumption and birthweight. How much drinking during pregnancy is safe? Journal of the American Medical Association 252:1875–1879

Mitchell J, Paiva M, Walker D, Heaton M 1999 BDNF and NGF afford in vitro neuroprotection against ethanol combined with acute ischaemia and chronic hypoglycaemia. Developmental Neuroscience 21(1):68–75

National Institute on Drug Abuse 1994 National Institute of Health statement of Alan I Leshner release of findings from NIDA's national pregnancy and health survey, Rockville, MD

Petrakis P 1987 Alcohol and birth defects: the fetal alcohol syndrome and related disorders. US Department of Health and Human Services, Public Health Service, Rockville, MD

Pietrantoni M, Knupple R 1991 Alcohol use in pregnancy. Clinical Perinatology 18(1):93–111

Queenan J, Hobbins J 1996 Protocols for high risk pregnancies. Blackwell Science, New York

Reckless W 1967 The crime problem. Appleton Century Crofts, New York

Reynolds K, Coombs D, Lowe J et al 1995 Evaluation of a self help program to reduce alcohol consumption among pregnant women. International Journal of the Addictions 30(4):427–443

Royal College of Obstetricians and Gynaecologists (RCOG) 1999 Alcohol consumption in pregnancy guideline. RCOG, London

Russell M, Martier S, Sokol R, Bottoms S, Jacobson S, Jacobson J 1994 Screening for pregnancy risk drinking. Alcoholism: Clinical and Experimental Research 18(5) (September/October):1156–1161

Serdula M, Williamson D, Kendrick J, Anda R, Byers T 1991 Trends in alcohol consumption by pregnant women: 1985–1988. Journal of the American Medical Association 265(7):876–879

Shen R, Hannigan J, Kapatos G 1999 Prenatal ethanol reduces the activity of adult mid brain dopamine neurons. Alcoholism: Clinical and Experimental Research 23(11):1801–1807

Smith I, Lancaster J, Moss-Wells S, Coles C, Falek A 1987 Identifying high risk pregnant drinkers: biological and behavioural correlates of continuous heavy drinking during pregnancy. Journal of Studies of Alcohol 48:304–309

Smith I E, Coles C D 1991 Multilevel intervention for prevention of fetal alcohol syndrome and effects of prenatal exposure. Recent Developments in Alcoholism 9:165–180

Smith K, Eckardt M 1991 The effects of prenatal alcohol on the central nervous system. Recent Developments in Alcoholism 9:151–164

Sokol R, Martier S 1996 Alcohol. In: Queenan J, Hobbins J (eds) Protocols for high risk pregnancies, 3rd edn. Blackwell Science, Cambridge, pp 675–688

Sokol R J, Martier S S, Ager J W 1989 The T-ACE questions: practical prenatal detection of risk-drinking. American Journal of Obstetrics and Gynecology 160:863–870

Stoler J, Holmes L 1999 Under-recognition of prenatal alcohol effects in infants of known alcohol abusing women. Comment. Journal of Pediatrics 135(4):405–406

Stratton K, Howe C, Battaglia F (eds) 1996 Institute of Medicine summary: fetal alcohol syndrome. National Academy Press, Washington DC

Streissguth A, Aase J, Clarren S et al 1991 Fetal alcohol syndrome in adolescents and adults. Journal of the American Medical Association 265(15):1961–1967

Tranmer J E 1985 Disposition of ethanol in maternal venous blood and the amniotic fluid. Journal of Obstetric, Gynaecological and Neonatal Nursing 14(6):484–490

Uhrich L 1997 Fetal alcohol syndrome and fetal alcohol effects and the role of childbirth educators in prevention. International Journal of Childbirth Education 12(3):25

US Surgeon General 1981 Surgeon General's advisory on alcohol and pregnancy. FDA Drug Bulletin. Food and Drug Administration, Rockville, MD 11:9–10

Walpole I, Zubrick S, Pontre J 1990 Is there a fetal effect with low to moderate alcohol use before or during pregnancy? Journal of Epidemiology and Community Health 44:297–301

Warren K R, Bast R J 1988 Alcohol related birth defects: an update. Public Health Reports 102(6):638–642

Waterson E, Murray-Lyon I 1989 Screening for alcohol related problems in the antenatal clinic: an assessment of different methods. Alcohol 24:21–30

Weiner L, Morse BA, Garrido P 1989 Fetal alcohol syndrome, fetal alcohol effect: focusing prevention on women at risk. International Journal of the Addictions 24(5):385–395

Wilsnack R, Wilsnack S 1992 Women, work and alcohol: failures of simple theories. Alcoholism: Clinical and Experimental Research 16:172–179

Wilsnack S, Klassen A, Schur B, Wilsnack R 1991 Predicting onset and chronicity of women's problem drinking: a five year longitudinal analysis. American Journal of Public Health 81(3):305–318

Recommended reading

Centres for Disease Control and Prevention 1998 Sociodemographic and behavioural characteristics associated with alcohol consumption during pregnancy – United States. Morbidity and Mortality Weekly Report 44:261–265

Exploration of factors associated with alcohol intake during pregnancy. An opportunity to tailor health promotion to individual needs.

Russell M, Martier S S, Sokol R J et al 1996 Detecting risk drinking during pregnancy: a comparison of four screening questionnaires. American Journal of Public Health 86(10):1435–1439

Investigation of the efficacy of screening for risk drinking behaviour during pregnancy, using several screening tools.

Exercise during pregnancy – a health option

8

Overview

Generally women are concerned with their own health and fitness and are increasingly taking part in regular exercise. It is therefore becoming more common for women who enter pregnancy to be engaged in some form of regular exercise and wish to continue this throughout pregnancy. The impact of appropriate preconception and antenatal education will enable women to make informed choices about partaking in or continuing exercise during pregnancy and ultimately influence lifestyle changes. Women who engage in exercise programmes have an opportunity to engage in midwifery-led exercise regimes, where they not only receive the physiological benefits of exercise during pregnancy, but benefit from social interaction with other pregnant women. Although anecdotal, my experience of leading aquanatal, antenatal and postnatal classes has reinforced my ideas of pregnancy motivating women toward making healthy lifestyle changes. Women who attended my aquanatal classes who had not exercised before, continued to do so beyond the postnatal period. This observation would benefit from controlled research investigation.

This chapter will examine the relative benefits and dangers of exercise during pregnancy with regards to the physiological adaptations to exercise stress, upon the physiological changes occurring as a result of pregnancy. Dynamic exercise which is concerned with muscular activity resulting in body movement will form the basis for discussion. Concepts of health and fitness are explored in relation to active exercise during pregnancy and safety measures are discussed. Prior knowledge and understanding of the following areas will enable the reader to understand the issues concerned with exercise during pregnancy highlighted in the chapter:

- the physiology of pregnancy
- fetal development
- risk management and risk assessment
- antenatal risk factors and their adverse effect on pregnancy.

What is exercise?

Exercise means different things to different people, but it is generally associated with fitness. Some people do not feel that they have exercised unless they have engaged in physical activity at a fitness gym. Others would consider for example; a brisk walk, yoga, relaxation, swimming, aerobics, stretch, squash, golf, or body conditioning as appropriate forms of exercise. Exercise is taken to mean any activity which involves promoting cardiovascular fitness, including aerobic work, either high impact, low impact or no impact work, muscular strength, muscular endurance and flexibility. Chamberlain & Pipkin (1998) suggest that any activity which involves lifting the body will inevitably be an extra cost in pregnancy owing to increasing body weight and therefore constitutes exercise.

People generally exercise to become fit or maintain fitness; the interpretation of this is varied. An outward appearance of well being is often confused with being healthy, the concept of which is discussed in Chapter 1. Health in its crudest sense is the absence of disease; it can therefore be postulated that one can be healthy without necessarily being fit. It is difficult, however, to be in a state of fitness without having a degree of good health. Physical fitness can be described as a state of health which enables the individual to partake in active exercise, without fatigue and with a sense of well being. Exercise is associated with feelings of psychological well being and increased self-esteem. Pregnancy in itself can be regarded as a form of exercise. The physiological changes during pregnancy are gradual and progressive. The body does not work each system harder than it is able, and self-disciplines and self-regulates to promote the health of the woman and her unborn baby. The joints are gently introduced to the increasing weight and the muscles work harder. This can be described as a training effect induced by weight gain. During pregnancy muscles work progressively harder; they adapt to the extra workload by becoming more efficient.

Changes during pregnancy – an overview

Most of the changes occurring during pregnancy are progressive and are due to either hormonal or physical alterations. The changes in blood volume, cardiac output, heart rate, systemic blood pressure, vascular resistance and distribution of blood flow are balanced by the maternal cardiovascular system to support the growing fetus and enable maternal tolerance.

Cardiovascular system

The cardiovascular system is challenged during pregnancy owing to an increased circulating blood mass, the placental circulating system, fetal nutritional requirements, the growing fetus adding to increase in body weight and increased levels of circulating oestrogen, progesterone and prostaglandin E_1 and E_2. The enlarging uterus causes an increase in intra-abdominal pressure, and a slight change in the position of the heart. This progressive alteration does not usually compromise the health of the mother. Exercise increases the demand of the cardiorespiratory system. If superimposed upon an existing health problem in which haemodynamics are already challenged, the maternal and fetal condition may be adversely affected. Risk assessment is an important starting point when discussing the continuation of exercise during pregnancy. It is not the remit of this chapter to detail physiological changes of the cardiovascular system during pregnancy, but in light of exercise demands the cardiovascular system deserves further attention.

During pregnancy, plasma represents 75% of the total blood volume increase. Progesterone and oestrogen mediate the increase of plasma renin activity and blood aldosterone levels. An increased level of plasma renin enhances sodium retention, which influences an increase in total body water. During pregnancy the vascular system has an increased distensibility, which influences the level of fluid retention. This is also influenced by the increased capacity of the uterine vein. The distribution of fluid is very often presented as ankle and foot oedema, but is primarily dependent on body position. An increase in venous capacitance contributes to vasodilatation at skin level, which increases heat loss, a valuable adjustment necessary to prevent hyperthermia during exercise. The resting heart rate increases by up to seven beats per minute in the first trimester and by 15 beats per minute in the second and third trimesters (Araujo 1997). It is suggested that those who perform endurance athletic activities can increase their performance during the first 12 to 15 weeks of pregnancy owing to increased blood volume and red cell mass functioning as an internal 'blood doping' system that has the potential to increase oxygen-carrying capacity (Clapp 1991).

Respiratory system

Major changes occur to the respiratory system which are mediated by mechanical, hormonal and biochemical changes.

The gradual increasing size of the uterus causes the resting position of the diaphragm to be raised by 4 centimetres above its natural rest position. Respiration is not compromised and the diaphragm accomplishes the major work of breathing, more so than the costal muscles. Due to the increased intra-abdominal pressure, the transverse diameter of the diaphragm increases by approximately 2 centimetres causing a flaring of the lower ribs. Pregnant women may experience an alteration in their normal breathing patterns, but they should not be automatically excluded or discouraged from continuing with exercise regimes carried out before pregnancy. The most important hormonal influences which cause changes to the respiratory system are mediated by prostaglandin and progesterone. Several theories suggest that circulating serum progesterone is an influencing factor. Circulating serum progesterone which gradually increases as pregnancy advances has been found to lower the carbon dioxide threshold of the respiratory centre, and causes increased sensitivity, which most likely contributes to feelings of dyspnoea (DeSwiet 1984). Another common theory is that progesterone causes water retention in the lung, which has a direct negative effect on the diffusion capacity. Hyperventilation follows in order to maintain normal PO_2 levels. In anticipation of major alterations it is suggested that progesterone reduces the resistance of the respiratory airways, thus enabling a greater flow of air and assisting breathing (Huch 1986). Changes in lung volumes, function and ventilation are also mediated by biochemical and mechanical factors, all of which indirectly help to support the growth of the fetus without compromising the woman's health. As pregnancy advances, oxygen consumption increases owing to increases in weight and body fat stores (ACOG 1994a).

Musculoskeletal system

Adaptation of the musculoskeletal system during pregnancy can affect the ability to exercise. The increase in progesterone and relaxin promotes joint laxity in preparation for delivery. The symphysis pubis and the sacroiliac joints soften. The woman's centre of gravity is changed owing to the anterior displacement of the enlarging uterus, which also exaggerates lumbar lordosis. Upper back and shoulder pain may occur owing to the enlarging heavy breasts, which can also affect the centre of gravity (Artal & Buckenmeyer 1995). Balance may be affected, hence it is useful to consider exercises which do not rely on a sense of balance during workout programmes.

Exercise during pregnancy – physiological considerations

During pregnancy the systems of the body go through major physiological changes to accommodate the demands of the growing fetus. It may be difficult to appreciate that physiological adaptations are adequate to provide for the combined demands of exercise and pregnancy. Regular sustained exercise is known to deplete carbohydrate stores, redistribute blood flow away from the splanchnic organs toward the working muscles and skin and induce a hyperthermia (Clapp 1995). Naturally, there may be concern about exercise during pregnancy and the effects on the fetus. The physiological changes induced by exercise during pregnancy stress the body system already challenged by pregnancy. Just as the maternal system copes with gradual progressive changes to cardiovascular and respiratory function, so too can the body maintain a healthy balance during exercise, with appropriate physiological adjustment in a healthy pregnancy. Numerous reports suggest that either continuing or beginning exercise during pregnancy has many positive effects and no negative effects on the pregnancy and outcome, when the pregnancy is progressing normally (Clapp 1991, Hatch, Shu & Mclean 1993, Wolfe, Brenner & Mottola 1994).

There is, however, a dearth of evidence from well-conducted double blind trials of exercise during pregnancy. This is primarily due to the ethical implications involved in asking pregnant women to engage in activities which have the potential to cause harm to the fetus. Many research studies discussed here are therefore based on animal subjects.

Circulation

During exercise the cardiac output increases with oxygen consumption and exercise intensity (Gilbert & Harman 1998). Studies have demonstrated that cardiac output increases to the same extent in pregnant women who exercise as in non-pregnant women engaging in the same level of exercise (Carpenter et al 1988, Sady et al 1989, 1990). During pregnancy, however, the increased cardiac output is thought to maintain the non-exercising vascular beds, primarily the uterus, placenta and ultimately the fetus (Sharp 1993). Exercise during pregnancy should not exceed the capacity of the cardiovascular system. This may be influenced by an increased duration of aerobic workout and excessive frequency. During exercise blood is diverted to the skin and skeletal muscles. Splanchnic and renal blood flows are reduced owing to vasoconstriction (Gilbert & Harman 1998). It is suggested that vasoconstriction varies depending on the severity of the exercise and can reduce blood flow by 80% (Queenan & Hobbins 1996). Blood flow to the brain and heart remain unchanged. If blood is

---

Discussion questions

- Which form of exercise do you consider to be safe during pregnancy?
- What factors have influenced your criteria for safety?
- What are the physiological concerns regarding the effects of exercise on the woman and fetus?
- Do you feel adequately prepared to discuss exercise issues during pregnancy?

diverted from the uterus, it may lead to acute fetal hypoxia and possible intrauterine growth retardation (Blackburn & Loper 1992). Overwhelming evidence suggests that this is unlikely. At rest over 50% of the entire cardiac output is directed toward the pelvic and abdominal viscera. During exercise a vasomotor-mediated vascular shunt reduces the cardiac output to these sites – by 21% (a fourfold increase in energy expenditure) during light exercise such as slow walking and 7% (a tenfold increase in energy expenditure) during moderate exercise such as jogging (Horvath 1979). Sharp (1993) questions whether the uterus is involved in the exercise-induced vascular shunt and concludes that, although uterine blood flow may diminish, oxygen delivery to the placenta and the uterus is virtually unchanged. During strenuous exercise, defined as 10 minutes at 70% maximum work, and very strenuous exercise, defined as 40 minutes at maximum work (exercising to the level where the rate of oxygen consumption cannot be further increased, $VO_{2\ max}$), animal studies have shown a marked reduction in uterine blood flow of 20%. Remarkably the oxygen uptake by the uterus remained unchanged. Lotgering, Gilbert & Longo (1983) suggest that this is a compensatory mechanism primarily resulting from haemoconcentration, blood flow which is selectively delivered to the cotyledons and an increased oxygen extraction by the uterus and its contents. Other animal studies suggest that at least 50% of uterine blood flow must be redistributed before there is any effect on the fetus. This is likely to happen only during overexhaustive, prolonged aerobic work (Wilkening & Meschia 1983).

Hypothermia

Basal body temperature rises by 0.5°C around the time of ovulation and reduces again only around the middle trimester of pregnancy, returning to preovulation levels. The amount of heat generated increases by 30–35% during pregnancy, predominantly due to fetoplacental metabolism (Blackburn & Loper 1992). In pregnancy, the body mass ratio to surface area alters, which has implications for heat exchange. However, peripheral vasodilatation with an increase in cutaneous blood flow and an increased activity of sweat glands promotes equilibrium. During exercise heat loss can be further influenced by environmental factors.

Fetal temperature is 0.5°C higher than that of the mother. The fetus cannot control its temperature independently, therefore heat from the metabolic activities of the fetus is dissipated through the amniotic fluid via the placenta to the maternal blood in the intervillous spaces. An efficient blood flow between heat exchange sites in the placenta is essential. During exercise body temperature will increase when heat production exceeds heat loss. Heat production during exercise is determined by the intensity, duration and efficiency of the exercise.

Strenuous prolonged exercise increases maternal core body temperature. Research carried out on animals suggests that the fetus can dissipate heat only when the maternal blood flow remains static. During exhaustive exercise there may be a reduction in uterine blood flow owing to demands from maternal muscle and skin (Speroff 1996), thus challenging the ability of the fetus to dissipate heat. Exercise to the point of exhaustion should therefore be avoided. Research on sheep highlighted an increased incidence of neural tube defects when the maternal core temperature was raised above 39°C during early pregnancy. It is also reported that the human neural tube is vulnerable to high temperatures during the first trimester of pregnancy; Sandford (1992) states that hot bath use increases the risk of spina bifida approximately 31-fold. Many women, however, may not know that they are pregnant during this time. Studies reported by Miller, Smith & Shepard (1978) conclude that probably 10% of 63 human pregnancies resulting in anencephalic babies had been associated with high temperature situations, and febrile illness during the first 5 weeks' gestation. The reported cases of febrile illness experienced temperatures of 38.9°C and above for approximately 3 days. There are to date no confirmed exercise-induced hyperthermic fetal malformations. Pregnant women are as equally well adapted as their non-pregnant counterparts to balancing heat production and heat loss (Khanna 1998). The risk of dehydration during exercise is increased, however; therefore hydration at this time is particularly important (Artal & Buckenmeyer 1995). Warm environments should be avoided when carrying out exercise whilst pregnant and attention paid to clothing which encourages heat loss.

Respiratory system

The increased sensitivity of the respiratory system to carbon dioxide has been highlighted above. This response occurs at rest and during exercise. During moderate exercise approximately 8 litres of air per minute are ventilated as opposed to 2 litres when the body is at rest (Sharp 1993). Minute ventilation increases with exercise intensity during pregnancy to eight times that of the resting value and compared with non-pregnant subjects it is significantly higher (Lotgering, Gilbert & Longo 1983). With increasing exercise intensity carbon dioxide levels rise. Hyperventilation that persists during exercise may be due to increased sensitivity of the respiratory system to carbon dioxide exhibited when at rest.

Metabolic changes

Pregnancy is a diabetogenic state characterised by mild fasting hypoglycaemia, postprandial hypoglycaemia and hyperinsulinemia. The rising levels of cortisol and progesterone during pregnancy predispose to carbohydrate intolerance by insulin resistance. Glucose clearance is therefore reduced. Such changes occur to ensure that the fetus receives adequate glucose levels (Queenan & Hobbins 1996). It is unlikely that a non-diabetic mother would induce a fetal hypoglycaemia during regular exercise. However Sharp (1993) states that exercising strenuously for an hour may cause significant lowering of blood glucose. Research carried out on non-diabetic pregnant rats clearly demonstrated hypoglycaemic effects on the fetus when exercising on a treadmill for 50 minutes, with rest phases (Treadway & Young 1991). The effects on humans are not well established.

During pregnancy 300 extra kilocalories a day are required to meet the metabolic demands (Araujo 1997). During regular exercise the calorific requirement is further increased with greater carbohydrate utilisation (Clapp et al 1988). Adequate intake of carbohydrates is thus essential for exercising pregnant women.

Fetal response to exercise

It is well documented that women who carried out strenuous exercise during pregnancy gained less weight, were more likely to deliver on or just before their due date (approximately 8 days) and delivered infants who had a consistently reduced birth weight compared with women who did not exercise during pregnancy (Artal, Dorey & Kirschbaum 1991, Clapp & Little 1995, McMurray et al 1993). Bell, Palma & Lumley (1995) established a link between vigorous exercise (exercise more than four times a week) and low birth weight. Evidence presented by Clapp & Capeless (1990) suggests that women who exercised more than four times a week had lower birth weight babies than their non-exercising counterparts. The reduction in birth weight was estimated to be approximately 500 g and was thought to be due to a reduction in fat mass. Kardel & Kase (1998), however, observed the effects of exercise on the fetus, which showed no compromise in fetal growth and development at high and medium intensity exercise and concluded that, if pregnancy is not compromised with adverse risk factors, exercise during pregnancy does not adversely affect birth weight.

Evidence suggesting that exercise during healthy pregnancy induces preterm labour is weak. Exercise induces an increase in adrenaline and serum noradrenaline. Adrenaline inhibits uterine activity whilst noradrenaline increases the amplitude and frequency of spontaneous uterine contractions. It is suggested that increasing levels of noradrenaline have the ability to cause uterine activity which begins preterm labour in women who are at increased risk (ACOG 1994b, Creasy 1994). Although there has been an association between strenuous physical work and an increased incidence of preterm labour, there is no assessment of recreational exercise and its effects on initiating preterm labour (Papiernik & Kaminiski 1974). Hatch et al (1998) sought to investigate the effect of vigorous exercise on the length of gestation and its association with preterm labour. Five hundred and fifty-seven antenatal women who performed heavy exercise (> 1000 kcal/week) were followed until the time of delivery. The results showed no association between heavy exercise and preterm labour. Heavy exercise was shown to reduce rather than raise the risk of preterm birth. Although noradrenaline increases during exercise, baseline uterine activity remains constant. If there is an increased risk of preterm labour during pregnancy, then recreational exercise should be avoided. Where preterm labour does not present itself as a risk factor, exercise does not increase its incidence. However, continuing vigorous exercise beyond this time reduces the chances of postmaturity (Clapp 1995).

There are no reports of fetal distress directly attributed to women who exercise. Variations in the fetal heart rate, however, have been reported. Maternal exercise causes fetal heart rate acceleration. The heart rate of the fetus can rise by 10 to 15 beats per minute after strenuous exercise, with reports of bradycardia occurring during the exercise. It is hypothesised that during times of bradycardia there is potential for periods of fetal hypoxia (Carpenter et al 1988). Although some authors report this to be a natural response experienced during exercise (Artal et al 1984) Rafla (1998) suggests that the fetus can tolerate brief periods of hypoxia and respond with tachycardia in a healthy pregnancy. This counteraction facilitates the circulation of blood to increase the oxygen supply. Bradycardia in the fetus during exercise and immediately after exercise has been associated with fitness levels of the mother. Wolfe, Brenner & Mottola (1994), found that 10 to 20 fetuses of unfit mothers (mothers who had not exercised before) experienced transient decreases in the heart rate during and immediately following moderate intensity and increasing intensity exercise. (Moderate exercise in this context was viewed as sustained cycle ergometry.) The results suggest that there is an increased risk of reduced uterine blood flow and fetal oxygen tension among the fetuses of women deemed as unfit who exercise at this level. No adverse fetal outcomes were presented. Observation of the fetus of low risk women during exercise and the fetus of women identified as high risk showed different fetal effects. In low risk pregnancies after exercise Rafla (1998) observed an increase in fetal heart rate from a mean of 143 beats per minute (bpm) to 148 bpm. In high risk pregnancies a transient decrease from 140 bpm to 141 bpm was observed. Ten cases of significant bradycardia were also noted in the high risk group following exercise. The bradycardia was thought to be indicative of fetal hypoxia. Current research studies have clearly shown that exercise is not harmful to the fetus in healthy pregnancies (Kardel & Kase 1998, Whitelaw & Rafla 1996). Adhering to safety parameters of exercise during pregnancy will enable physiological adjustment to take place safely without compromise to the woman and fetus. Gentle warm-up and careful attention paid to the length of aerobic workout is therefore essential. Women should be discouraged from working through pain, and working to excessive breathlessness.

Aquanatal exercises

Due to the increases in body weight during pregnancy women may find exercise in water extremely useful. Water has been used for centuries to relieve pain and promote muscular relaxation. The physiological effects of immersion and exercise also have many benefits. Exercise in water is relatively a non-weight-bearing activity and would be beneficial to those women who have not exercised before but wish to start exercising during pregnancy. Water can be used for support or resistance so that muscles can work harder without causing joint damage. It is becoming increasingly common for midwives to lead aquanatal classes, which in itself provides rewards and benefits for women who have a professional on tap to offer advice and support about pregnancy, labour and parenting issues. Also relaxation, breathing and pelvic floor exercises can be incorporated into classes led by midwives. Exercise in water minimises the risk of injury.

Physiological changes during immersion include hydrostatic pressure, buoyancy and upthrust. Water exerts hydrostatic pressure on the surface of the body underwater, equal to the density of the water. Hydrostatic pressure exerts a force which pushes extravascular fluid into the vascular space, resulting in increased plasma volume by 4–6%; this in turn initiates diuresis. Diuresis peaks within 1 hour after the exercise class, with urine flow returning to normal after approximately 4 hours. The volume of diuresis correlates with the level of oedema. Research suggests that after immersion of 20 to 40 minutes during pregnancy there is a 300–400 ml loss of fluid, with blood volume being maintained (Mittlemark & Drinkwater 1992). The resistance of water around the chest wall improves respiratory function. The hydrokinetic effect of immersion in water gives a sensation of the abolition of gravity. Humans have a specific gravity of less than one and will therefore float. Archimedes' principle states that a body at rest which is wholly or partly immersed in a fluid experiences an upthrust that is equal to the weight of the fluid displaced. Thus the feeling of weighing less when in water gives the buoyancy effect.

Psychological benefits

The psychological benefits of regular exercise during pregnancy include improved self-esteem and self-image. Generally those who engage in regular exercise are motivated toward improving self-image and often enjoy the physiological benefits of regular exercise. Exercise minimises the minor discomforts associated with pregnancy, prepares the body for labour and speeds postpartum physical recovery (Zeanah & Schlosser 1993). Although placebo effects could be a contributory factor to such positive responses, Horns et al (1996) demonstrated similar findings and concluded that women who engaged in active exercise had fewer of the common discomforts associated with pregnancy. However, pregnancy may have a positive psychological effect in itself which may increase self-esteem. A well-established cause of increased self-esteem after exercise is the release of beta endorphins, which are morphine analogues, into tissue during exercise; these not only have analgesic action but also enhance personal feelings of well being. Pregnant women who engage in physical exercise, particularly in scheduled programmes designed for pregnant mothers to be, will inevitably benefit from social interaction with others, which may lead to building social networks, sharing ideas and problems and therefore create a feeling of well being. Without adequate controls, therefore, research assessing the results of exercise on maternal psychological well being should be viewed with caution.

Consideration of safety aspects

The midwife is very often viewed by pregnant clients as the health professional with expert knowledge on all aspects related to pregnancy and childbirth. Although this is not entirely the case, the provision of clear, current research-based evidence can enable midwives to advise women about their existing or proposed exercise regimes. The following points may provide useful tips and advice for midwives to incorporate in discussion about exercise during pregnancy:

- Exercise instruction must be carried out by professionally trained personnel by an approved institution.
- Maximal recommended heart rate is estimated by subtracting the subject's age from 220 (Rafla 1998).
- Review the aims of participation in exercise: exercise should be directed toward the maintenance of good posture and improved body awareness.
- Fitness instructors generally begin exercises classes by establishing the pregnancy status of the group; if omitted it is the woman's responsibility to highlight this.
- A woman who presents with any risk markers after risk assessment should not be encouraged to exercise (please refer to previous definition of exercise) unless written advice is received from her obstetrician.
- Women who have not engaged in regular exercise before and wish to do so during pregnancy should not be discouraged (if they do not present with adverse risk factors). Participating in exercise during pregnancy will inevitably improve their fitness.

- If asked to suggest a form of exercise for those women who have not exercised before, you may suggest an appropriate aquanatal class. This will promote the comfort of exercise in water, which provides added benefits of buoyancy and upthrust, thus reducing pressure on muscles and joints without stressed physical impact.
- Remember, it is essential to highlight that exercise done incorrectly can lead to injury, especially during pregnancy.

The American College of Obstetricians and Gynecologists (ACOG) issued guidelines in 1985 (ACOG 1994b) to ensure the safety of pregnant women taking exercise. Whilst providing safety parameters and guidance for health promotion work, they were restrictive, particularly for women who started their pregnancies with increased cardiorespiratory fitness. With further developments and published research on exercise during pregnancy, the guidelines have been revised. The current guidelines are less didactic and enable flexibility and range when planning exercise programmes. The following is a summary of the current guidelines which have been derived from a critical analysis of the available physiological data regarding exercise and pregnancy and are intended for those women who have no risk factors (ACOG 1994b).

1. During pregnancy women can continue to exercise at mild to moderate levels regularly (at least three times a week). This is preferable to intermittent activity.
2. Women should avoid exercising in the supine position and avoid prolonged periods of motionless standing.
3. Pregnant women should stop exercising when fatigued and not exercise to exhaustion.
4. Weight-bearing exercises may be continued under certain circumstances, but should be maintained at intensities similar to prepregnancy and not increased.
5. Non-weight-bearing exercises reduce the risk of injury and facilitate the continuation of exercise during pregnancy.
6. Exercise which poses a risk of abdominal trauma should be avoided.
7. Women who exercise should ensure they take an adequate diet.
8. During the first trimester attention should be paid to enhancing heat loss through appropriate clothing, adequate hydration and optimal environmental conditions.
9. Postpartum exercise should be resumed gradually and determined by the woman's physical capability.

Reflection point

- Reflect on the questions you have asked about antenatal exercise. In light of the ACOG guidelines, what advice would you offer about exercise during pregnancy?

Causes for concern

Pregnant women should be advised to avoid exercise and sport activities which may cause harm to themselves during pregnancy or pose a risk to the fetus. Contact sports pose a risk of trauma and are not advisable, or any sports which present the potential risk of trauma to the woman and fetus.

Consideration must be given to concerns about redistribution of weight, increased cardiac workload, hypothermia and hormonal influences. Sports employing jogging, jumpy, or jerky rapid movements should be practised with caution. During pregnancy impact exercise is inadvisable as it poses additional stress on the pelvic floor and joints which are already affected by pregnancy hormones. Deep flexion or extension of joints must be avoided because of joint instability invoked by the pregnancy hormones relaxin and progesterone. Care should also be taken during low impact work such as side steps and knee bends for the same reason. Extra care and attention is needed if unilateral leg movements are used. There is an increased need for stability during exercise and as such unilateral leg movement invokes an uneven distribution of weight within the pelvic girdle, which would cause stress on the sacroiliac joints and symphysis pubis. Stretching to increase flexibility during pregnancy should be avoided (Baddeley 1999). However, short static stretches may be useful during relaxation exercise where the aim is to relieve tension.

Deep working of the abdominus rectus muscles must be avoided, as this muscle is stretched and weakened during pregnancy. However, attention to strengthening the muscle to help maintain good posture and support the lower back can be carried out without practising curl-up sit-up exercises. Also exercise in the supine position should be avoided, as this would compromise blood flow to the fetus. The compression of the inferior vena cava by the uterus late in gestation (i.e. more than 24 weeks) results in decreased venous return and a marked decrease in cardiac output. The heavy gravid uterus applies pressure to the blood flow through the inferior vena cava. Research evidence has identified a 20% fall in uterine blood flow during strenuous supine exercise. Women should be discouraged from partaking in exercise which encourages a Valsalva manoeuvre. The compromise to the fetus may present as varying degrees of hypoxia and predispose to fetal distress (Artal & Buckenmeyer 1995).

Social exclusion

People living on low incomes are not always able to make choices about taking part in exercise programmes. The provision of such services frequently takes place within facilities which may, by the very nature of the location and the idealistic fitness culture, exclude socioeconomically disadvantaged members of the community. Other barriers to participation include financial implications, poor accessibility and poor childcare provision. Efforts to make exercise fitness environments available and accessible to meet the needs of the socioeconomically disadvantaged groups may encourage participation and help reduce social exclusion. Social exclusion has been shown to have negative effects on health. Kawachi et al (1996) found that people who were socially isolated were three times more likely to commit suicide than people who had good social support including numerous social ties. In addition to the physiological benefits of exercise during pregnancy, the environment provides an opportunity for social interaction. Exercise programmes specifically organised for pregnant women provide an excellent opportunity for women to share information and offer support to each other, to the point of building networks which provide social support. Machin & Scamell (1998) highlighted that women who do not attend antenatal education classes depend heavily on friendship networks for their information, advice and support. The government white paper Our healthier nation, a contract for health (Secretary of State for Health 1998) recognises that exercise is an excellent way of fostering good health and a healthy lifestyle and the importance of promoting fitness by exercise. This national contract for health states that health professionals should provide sound information and advice on the health risks resulting from lack of exercise. The proposal for healthy-living centres will be of particular relevance for those people who have been excluded from the opportunities to achieve better health through exercise. The government proposes that they will establish a health link in the most deprived areas for those who perceive existing health and fitness centres 'off-putting or difficult to get to'. Midwives' influence in supporting women to continue exercise regimens throughout pregnancy, or begin safe exercise during pregnancy should not be undervalued and forms part of the national strategy to improve health.

The pelvic floor and health

Urinary incontinence – a legacy of childbirth?

The pelvic floor has an important and extensive function and awareness of this forms a major part of women's health education. It functions as a support for the abdominal and pelvic organs, assists in the mechanism of labour, allows the control for urine and faeces and has a sexual function. The bladder is under increasing stress during pregnancy and childbirth, hence overdistension and trauma should be avoided. Although it is thought that epidural anaesthesia has a protective effect in relaxing the pelvic floor during childbirth, it is, however, also associated with retention of urine. Immediately postdelivery there is an increased diuresis lasting up to approximately 8 to 10 hours. Women who have used the epidural for pain relief may not feel the sensation of a full bladder for some several hours postdelivery as bladder sensation is the last sensation to be regained. The midwife's vigilance during labour and the immediate postpartum period reduces the risk of urinary problems occurring. During pregnancy and childbirth, however, the pelvic floor muscles are placed under increased stress, which in severe cases if undetected or left untreated may lead to immediate urinary problems and prolapse of pelvic organs during later life.

Women are therefore encouraged to perform pelvic floor exercises during the antenatal and postpartum period. Education is also directed toward the continuation of pelvic floor exercise beyond pregnancy and childbirth to form part of routine daily activities. During general exercise, as described in the previous sections, the pelvic floor becomes slightly toned. However, attention should also be paid toward specific pelvic floor exercises. Conclusive evidence to support the benefits of pelvic floor exercises in the prevention of, or amelioration of, urinary incontinence is limited, although there is some evidence to suggest that performing pelvic floor exercises particularly in the antenatal period has some protective effect (Keane 1997, Wilson, Herbison & Herbison 1996). Exercises aimed at strengthening the pelvic floor are therefore still advocated.

During antenatal education and/or preconception classes the midwife should use the opportunity to explore the sensitive subject of urinary incontinence. This is considered by many to be a shameful socially unacceptable condition which is difficult to communicate and seek help about. Older ideas of incontinence during pregnancy and following childbirth considered the dysfunction to be a normal consequence of giving birth. Seeking help for what was considered to be a taboo subject was virtually unheard of. Today, however, attitudes of the public and the health professional's responsibility have changed dramatically. Seeking clarity when asking questions about urine and bowel function has significant health benefits. Scowen (1996) states that asking if a woman's urine and bowel function are 'normal' is ineffective communication. This is because perceptions of normal are influenced by life experiences and, as such, mothers and grandmothers who have experienced incontinence and coped by themselves may view this as a natural consequence of childbirth (Scowen 1996). Exploring and challenging such ideas during antenatal education can help to reduce existing social and cultural barriers, provide a vehicle for free discussion and ultimately increase the level of help sought.

Urinary incontinence is defined by the International Continence Society (1997) as, 'a condition in which involuntary loss of urine is a social or hygienic problem and is objectively demonstrable'. It affects one in four of the adult female population (Herbert 1998). The most common type of urinary incontinence in women is stress incontinence. This is defined as the involuntary loss of urine during coughing, sneezing or physical exertion (Dawson & Whitfield 1996). The symptoms sometimes develop during pregnancy or after delivery and are thought to be a result of weakness of the pelvic floor muscles caused by stretching during pregnancy and delivery. Whether it is pregnancy or delivery which predisposes to urinary incontinence is a controversial discussion topic (Wilson, Herbison & Herbison 1996). Studies of urethral and anal sphincter electrophysiology indicate that it may be the process of vaginal delivery that predisposes to urinary incontinence as damage to the pudendal nerve may occur during the delivery process, resulting in subsequent denervation of the striated muscle of the pelvic floor and urethra (Smith, Hosker & Warrell 1989, Snooks et al 1985).

Research evidence suggests that the symptoms of urinary incontinence commonly develop during or following delivery and are more common among multiparous women (Jolleys 1988). It is likely that multiparity adversely affects the function of the pelvic floor, indeed Thomas et al (1980) purport that parity of four or more has been associated with urinary incontinence, more so than the mode of delivery. It is difficult to conclude, however, that the mode of delivery bears no relation to the integrity of the pelvic floor. Jolleys (1988) found some correlation between perineal suturing and incontinence. The cause of perineal trauma was not determined, but could be classified as a contributory factor – for example, previous third degree tear, prolonged second stage of labour and fetal distress resulting in episiotomy. A study exploring the association between caesarean section, obesity and parity, with the prevalence of urinary incontinence, 3 months after delivery was able to exclude caesarean section as a predisposing factor. Parity and obesity were identified as significant risk factors (Wilson et al 1996).

Urinary incontinence has also been found in women who have never had children, which suggests that the causes are not always related to childbirth (Scowen 1996). Thirty-one per cent of childless women under the age of 25 have suffered from urinary incontinence (Jolleys 1988). Plausible explanations suggest that the altered neurological function and collagen content of the pelvic soft tissues may point toward a genetic disposition (Churchill et al 1994, De Groat 1990, Nordling 1990). Definite causes, however, remain unclear.

Teaching isolated muscle pelvic floor exercises

Muscle fibres which make up the pelvic floor are both slow twitch and fast twitch muscles. It is essential to encourage women to exercise both muscle fibres in order for the pelvic floor to be exercised effectively (see Box 8.1). Slow twitch muscle fibres are designed to work for long periods of time without fatigue. The majority of the pelvic floor muscle is made up of slow twitch muscle fibres (70%), because they are necessary to support the pelvic contents. The levator ani muscles (deep layer of the pelvic floor), are made of fast twitch muscle. They react quickly to changes in abdominal pressure, for example during coughing and sneezing. Fast twitch muscle

Box 8.1 **Case study: Rose**

Rose is 37 years old and is pregnant for the fourth time. She has had three previous normal vaginal deliveries. During a routine antenatal visit Rose informs the midwife that she finds it difficult to conduct pelvic floor exercises because of a urine infection. Each time she attempts to exercise her pelvic floor the pain experienced when trying to pass urine stops her. She asks the midwife for advice.

Reflection points

- When does Rose conduct pelvic floor exercises?
- What is wrong with her technique and why?
- What should the midwife advise?

fibres produce short bursts of energy and are easily fatigued (Thompson 1999).

To exercise both types of muscle fibre there needs to be a combination of exercises that are performed quickly and slowly. First, identification of the pelvic floor is essential, as it should not be assumed that women automatically know where the pelvic floor is located. Visual representation of this area, using a clear diagram, would be useful. Discussing and exploring the functions of the pelvic floor and its role during childbirth will also enhance the learning process and help clients to recognise the need to exercise it. Sometimes, even after clear teaching and discussion on how to perform the exercise, accurate compliance is not guaranteed. Bump et al (1991) found that after teaching the exercise some women were unable to contract the pelvic floor muscles, but instead performed a Valsalva manoeuvre, or contraction of the gluteal and thigh muscles. Herbert (1998) suggests that there are two check systems which could ensure compliance. Either women can be asked to stop and start the flow of urine to locate the pelvic floor area only (this technique should not be used to exercise the pelvic floor, see Box 8.1), or they can place two fingers on the perineal area, and contract the muscle; if the muscle raises away from the fingers the exercise is deemed to be performed correctly. Motivation to perform pelvic floor exercises may be difficult when in practice the exercises are carried out in isolation with little perceived benefit by the woman. Indeed, evidence suggests that lack of motivation, ambivalence about the belief that the exercises work and social isolation when performing pelvic floor exercises are major causes of non-compliance (Ashworth & Hagan 1993).

Efficacy of pelvic floor exercises

Arnold Kegel (1948) proposed the use of pelvic floor exercises in the 1940s to strengthen the pelvic floor muscles after childbirth, to treat urinary stress incontinence and correct mild anatomical defects. A cure rate of 84% was presented. More recently, a study compared the effect of pelvic floor exercises, electrical stimulation, vaginal cones and no treatment

Box 8.2 **Pelvic Floor exercises**

Women should be encouraged to find their own starting points, by recording the number of contractions performed before the muscles are fatigued. This will be used as a baseline for improvement of endurance and strength. Exercises may start at eight contractions of both exercises 5 times a day, and progress to 10 contractions of both exercises eight times a day, and so on.

Advice may be, for example:

Squeeze and lift the pelvic floor and hold for 10 seconds. Repeat this contraction 10 times. Remember to hold for 10 seconds each time.

or:

Squeeze or pinch your back passage (anus) together as though you are stopping yourself from passing wind. Likewise squeeze your front passage (urethra) together as though you are stopping the flow of urine. Lift both up together and hold for 10 seconds. Repeat 10 times, remembering to hold for 10 seconds each time.

next:

Squeeze and lift the pelvic floor and release, repeat for 10.

or:

Squeeze or pinch your back passage (anus) together as though you are stopping yourself from passing wind. Likewise squeeze your front passage (urethra) together as though you are stopping the flow of urine. Lift both up together and then release.

for genuine stress incontinence. The results showed that improvement in muscle strength was significantly greater ($P = 0.03$) after pelvic floor exercises. The researcher concluded that training of the pelvic floor muscle is superior to electrical stimulation and vaginal cones in the treatment of stress incontinence (Bo, Talseth & Holme 1999).

Pelvic floor exercises involve voluntary contraction and relaxation of the levator ani muscles. Box 8.2 demonstrates the principles of Kegel pelvic muscle exercises. Once clients understand the functions and position of the pelvic floor and how to test the accuracy of the exercise, the exercise regimen detailed in Box 8.2 can be followed.

Summary

- Women naturally seek advice and support from the midwife about the safety of their exercise routines and potential harm to themselves and the fetus.
- Regular exercise, if carried out safely, provides both short and long term benefits to the woman and fetus. Encouraging and supporting

women to continue or start exercise which is considered safe during pregnancy requires knowledge and understanding of the physiological effects of exercise during pregnancy.

- Most of the changes occurring during pregnancy are progressive and are due to either hormonal or physical alterations.
- Cardiac output increases to the same extent in pregnant women who exercise as in non-pregnant women engaging in the same level of exercise. Exercise during pregnancy should not exceed the capacity of the cardiovascular system.
- Levels of continuing exercise will be determined by the woman's risk status and her present level of fitness.
- During exercise blood is diverted to the skin and skeletal muscles; uterine blood flow may diminish; oxygen delivery to the placenta and the uterus is virtually unchanged.
- Pregnant women are as equally well adapted as their non-pregnant counterparts to balancing heat production and heat loss. Attention should be paid to hydration needs and the environmental temperature, which may impede insensible heat loss.
- Midwives should be aware of the risks of exercise to the woman and fetus so that appropriate advice can be given. Adhering to safety parameters of exercise during pregnancy will enable physiological adjustment to take place safely without compromise to the woman and fetus.
- Where preterm labour does not present as a risk factor, exercise does not increase the incidence of preterm labour prior to $37^{1}/_{2}$ weeks' gestation.
- During pregnancy, impact exercise is inadvisable as it poses additional stress on the pelvic floor and joints which are already affected by pregnancy hormones. Women should be discouraged from partaking in exercise which encourages a Valsalva manoeuvre. The compromise to the fetus may present as varying degrees of hypoxia and predispose to fetal distress.
- In the absence of obstetric and medical risk factors pregnant women can exercise safely during pregnancy. Exercise programmes should be geared to suit the individual needs of the woman but guided by evidence-based guidelines.
- The woman should be informed of the potential risks associated with exercise during pregnancy so that she can make informed decisions about her programme. Jumpy, jerky, rapid movements (impact work) should be practised with caution, and impact exercise and deep flexion or extension of joints must be avoided.
- Childbirth and urinary incontinence are inextricably linked. Antenatal pelvic floor exercises and caesarean section have been shown to give

some protection of the pelvic floor from urinary incontinence, but this is not complete. Pelvic floor exercises should be encouraged and taught from a practical perspective to ensure that muscles are exercised appropriately.

References

American College of Obstetrians and Gynecologogists (ACOG) 1994a Exercise during pregnancy and the postpartum period. International Journal of Obstetrics and Gynecology 45:65–70

American College of Obstetrians and Gynecologogists (ACOG) 1994b Exercise during pregnancy and the postpartum period, technical bulletin no 189. ACOG, Washington DC

Araujo D 1997 Expecting questions about exercise and pregnancy. The Physician and Sportsmedicine 25(4):85–93

Artal R, Buckenmeyer P J 1995 Exercise during pregnancy and postpartum. Contemporary Obstetrics and Gynaecology (May):62–72

Artal R et al 1984 Fetal bradycardia induced by maternal exercise. Lancet ii:258

Artal R, Dorey F J, Kirschbaum T A 1991 Effect of maternal exercise on pregnancy outcome. In: Artal M R, Wiswell R A, Drinkwater B (eds) Exercise in pregnancy, 2nd edn. Williams & Wilkins, Baltimore MD, pp 213–224

Ashworth P D, Hagan M T 1993 Some social consequences of non compliance with pelvic floor exercises. Physiotherapy 79(7):465–470

Baddeley S 1999 Health-related fitness during pregnancy. Quay Books, Salisbury, Wiltshire

Bell R J, Palma S M, Lumley J M 1995 The effect of vigorous exercise during pregnancy on birth weight. Australian and New Zealand Journal of Obstetrics and Gynaecology 35:46–51

Blackburn S T, Loper L L 1992 Maternal, fetal, and neonatal physiology: a clinical perspective. W B Saunders, Mexico

Bo K, Talseth T, Holme I 1999 Single blind, randomised controlled trial of pelvic floor exercises, electrical stimulation, vaginal cones, and no treatment in management of genuine stress incontinence in women. British Medical Journal 318 (February)

Bump R C, Hurt G, Fantl A, Wyman J 1991 Assessment of Kegal pelvic muscle exercise performance after brief verbal instruction. American Journal of Obstetrics and Gynecology 163(92):322–329

Carpenter M W, Sady S S, Hoegsherp B et al 1988 Fetal heart rate response to maternal exhaustion. Journal of the American Medical Association 59(20):3006

Chamberlain G, Pipkin F 1998 Clinical physiology in obstetrics. Blackwell Science, Oxford

Churchill B M, Gilmore R F, Jayanthi V R et al 1994 Loss of elasticity in dysfunctional bladders: urodynamic and histochemical correlation. Journal of Urology 152:702–705

Clapp J F 1991 The changing thermal response to exercise during pregnancy. American Journal of Obstetrics and Gynecology 165:1684–1689

Clapp J F 1995 The interaction between regular exercise and selected aspects of women's health. American Journal of Obstetrics and Gynecology 173(1)

Clapp J F, Capeless E L 1990 Neonatal morphometrics after endurance exercise during pregnancy. American Journal of Obstetrics and Gynecology 163:1805–1811

Clapp J F, Little K 1995 The interaction between regular exercise and selected aspects of women's health. American Journal of Obstetrics and Gynecology 173(1):2–9

Clapp J F, Seaward B L, Sleamaker R H, Hiser J 1988 Maternal physiological adaptations to early human pregnancy. American Journal of Obstetrics and Gynecology 159:1456–1460

Creasy R 1994 Preterm labour and delivery. In: Creasy R, Resnick R (eds) Maternal-fetal medicine: principles and practice. W B Saunders, Philadelphia

Dawson C, Whitfield H 1996 Urinary incontinence and urinary infection. British Medical Journal 312.961–964

De Groat W C 1990 Central neural control of the lower urinary tract, neurobiology of incontinence. Ciba Foundation symposium. John Wiley, Chichester

DeSwiet M 1984 Maternal pulmonary disorders. In: Creasy R, Resnik R (eds) Maternal-fetal medicine: principles and practice. W B Saunders, Philadelphia

Gaskell J 1992 Exercise in pregnancy. Journal of the Association of Chartered Physiotherapists in Obstetrics and Gynaecology 73:5–7

Gilbert E, Harman J 1998 High risk pregnancy and delivery. Mosby, New York

Hatch C M, Shu X O, Mclean D E 1993 Maternal exercise during pregnancy, physical fitness and fetal growth. American Journal of Epidemiology 137:1105–1114

Hatch M, Levin B, Shu X O, Susser M 1998 Maternal leisure-time exercise and timely delivery. American Journal of Public Health 88(10):1528–1533

Herbert J 1998 Overcoming the pelvic flaw: exercise for continence. Professional Care of Mother and Child 8(2):39–41

Horns P, Ratcliffe L, Leggett J, Swanson M 1996 Pregnancy outcomes among active and sedentary primiparous women. Journal of Obstetric, Gynaecological and Neonatal Nursing Clinical Studies 25(1):49–54

Horvath S M 1979 Influence of differing intensity of exercise on blood flow distribution. Diabetes 28 (suppl):33–38

Huch R 1986 Maternal ventilation and the fetus. Journal of Perinatology 13:3

International Continence Society 1997 First international conference for the prevention of incontinence. Consensus statement. The Continence Foundation, London

Jolleys J V 1988 Reported prevalence of urinary incontinence in women in a general practice. British Medical Journal 296:1300–1302

Kardel K R, Kase T 1998 Training in pregnant women: effects on fetal development and birth. American Journal of Obstetrics and Gynecology 178(2):280–286

Kawachi I, Colditz G A, Ascherio A et al 1996 A prospective study of social networks in relation to total mortality and cardiovascular disease in men in the USA. Journal of Epidemiology and Community Health 50:245–251

Keane D 1997 Can incontinence after pregnancy be prevented? Pulse (November 29):69–70

Kegel A 1948 Progressive resistance exercise in the functional restoration of the perineal muscles. American Journal of Obstetrics and Gynecology 56:242–245

Khanna H 1998 Effects of exercise on pregnancy. American Family Physician 57(9):1770–1772

Lotgering F K, Gilbert R D, Longo L D 1983 Exercise responses in pregnant sheep: oxygen consumption, uterine blood flow and blood volume. Journal of Applied Physiology 55:834–841

Machin D, Scamell A 1998 Using ethnographic research to examine effects of 'informed choice'. British Journal of Midwifery 6(5):304–309

McMurray R G, Mottola M F, Wolfe L A et al 1993 Recent advances in understanding maternal and fetal responses to exercise. Medicine and Science in Sports and Exercise 25:1305–1321

Miller P, Smith D W, Shepard T N 1978 Maternal hyperthermia as a possible cause of anencephaly. Lancet 1:481–484

Mittlemark R A, Drinkwater B 1992 Exercise in pregnancy. Williams & Wilkins, Baltimore, MD

Nordling J 1990 Functional assessment of the bladder, neurobiology of incontinence. Ciba Foundation symposium 151. John Wiley, Chichester, pp 139–147

Papiernik E, Kaminiski M 1974 Multifactorial study of the risk of prematurity at 32 weeks of gestation. Journal of Perinatal Medicine 2:30–36

Queenan J T, Hobbins J C 1996 Protocols for high risk pregnancies. Blackwell Science, New York

Rafla N M 1998 The effect of maternal exercise on fetal heart action. Contemporary Reviews in Obstetrics and Gynaecology 10(3):171–176

Sady S P, Carpenter M W, Thompson P D, Sady M A, Haydon B, Coustan D R 1989 Cardiovascular response to cycle exercise during and after pregnancy. Journal of Applied Physiology 66:336–341

Sady M A, Haydon B B, Sady S P, Carpenter M W, Thompson P D, Coustan D R 1990 Cardiovascular response to maximal cycle exercise during pregnancy and at two and seven months postpartum. American Journal of Obstetrics and Gynecology 162:1181–1185

Sandford M K 1992 Neural tube defect etiology: new evidence concerning maternal hypothermia, health and diet. Developmental Medicine and Child Neurology 34:661–675

Scowen P 1996 Childbirth and continence: 2. Report on the 'your baby, your bladder, your bowels' conference held to mark National Continence Day, 1996. Professional Care of Mother and Child 6(5):119–122

Secretary of State for Health 1998 Our healthier nation, a contract for health. A consultation paper. The Stationery Office, London

Sharp C 1993 Physiological aspects of pregnancy and exercise. Journal of the Association of Chartered Physiotherapists in Obstetrics and Gynaecology 73(August):8–13

Smith A R B, Hosker G L, Warrell D W 1989 The role of pudendal nerve damage in the aetiology of genuine stress incontinence in women. British Journal of Obstetrics and Gynaecology 96:29–32

Snooks S J, Swash M, Henry M M, Setchell M 1985 Risk factors in childbirth causing damage to the pelvic floor innervation. British Journal of Surgery 72(suppl):S15–S17

Speroff L 1996 Exercise. In: Queenan T, Hobbins J (eds) Protocols for high risk pregnancies. Blackwell Science, New York, pp 42–50

Thomas T, Plymat K, Blannin J, Meade T 1980 Prevalence of urinary incontinence. British Medical Journal 281:1243–1245

Thompson J 1999 Incontinence in adults and children: part 2. Community Practitioner 72(4):96–97

Treadway J, Young A C 1991 Decreased glucose uptake in the fetus after maternal exercise. Medicine and Science in Sports and Exercise 22(2):140–145

Whitelaw N L, Rafla N M 1996 The effect of maternal exercise on fetal aortic blood flow. Journal of Obstetrics and Gynaecology 16:342–346

Wilkening R B, Meschia G 1983 Fetal oxygen uptake, oxygenation and acid-base balance as a function of uterine blood flow. American Journal of Physiology 244:H749

Wilson P D, Herbison R M, Herbison G P 1996 Obstetric practice and the prevalence of urinary incontinence three months after delivery. British Journal of Obstetrics and Gynaecology 103:154–161

Wolfe L A, Brenner I K M, Mottola M F 1994 Maternal exercise, fetal well being and pregnancy outcome. Exercise and Sports Science 22:145–194

Zeanah M, Schlosser S P 1993 Adherence to ACOG guidelines on exercise during pregnancy: effect on pregnancy outcome. Journal of Obstetric, Gynaecological and Neonatal Nursing 22:329–335

Recommended reading

Baddeley S 1999 Health related fitness during pregnancy. Quay Books, Salisbury, Wiltshire

Provision of basic guidelines on physical activity during pregnancy, including physiological adaptation to exercise during pregnancy.

Clapp J F 1998 The one year morphometric and neurodevelopment outcome of the offspring of women who continued to exercise regularly throughout pregnancy. American Journal of Obstetrics and Gynecology 178(23):594–599

Research which examines the morphometric and neurodevelopment outcome of offspring whose mothers exercise throughout pregnancy.

Clapp J F, Capeless E 1992 The $VO_{2\ max}$ of recreational athletes before and after pregnancy. Medicine and Science in Sports and Exercise 23(10):1128–1133

Mittelmark R A, Posner M D 1991 Fetal responses to maternal exercise. In: Mittlemark R A, Wiswell R A, Drinkwater B L (eds) Exercise in pregnancy, 2nd edn. Williams & Wilkins, Baltimore MD

Mental health promotion – a challenge for midwives

9

Overview

The World Health Organization's definition of health implies that there can be a complete state of mental health. The difficulties implicit when defining complete states of health have been explored in Chapter 1. It is logical to imply that mental well being is maintained when facets of an individual's personal ideas of social, physical, emotional, spiritual, societal and environmental health are challenged. Individual response to challenge is varied and is largely determined by cultural influence and social circumstance at the time of exposure. Mental health problems continue to be a major cause of ill health and are a significant predisposing risk factor for many physical health problems (Prescott-Clarke & Primatesta 1997). This chapter seeks to explore mental ill health from two perspectives, which have relevance to midwifery practice. The first part is concerned with postnatal depression aetiology, prevalence detection and screening. A clear emphasis on health education and social support is a prominent health promotion strategy within this section. The second part is concerned with post-traumatic stress disorder of survivors of rape and sexual assault. The long term sequelae of these experiences may be so profound that experiences of pregnancy and childbirth uncover the problems associated with the disorder. Integral to this section is the reality of mental trauma and its association with physical illness.

Postnatal depression

The postnatal period involves both physical and psychological adjustment to parenthood. Feelings of excitement, intrigue, responsibility and a sense of accomplishment are very often coupled with feelings of uncertainty, anxiety and in some cases self-doubt. Careful planning and preparation during the antenatal period cannot totally prepare women for the impact that motherhood will have on their everyday lives. The birth of the baby often presents a reality that is both emotionally and physically challenging for the woman and her partner.

During the postnatal period the woman is left with the legacy of postpartum physical discomfort and reflections of pregnancy and the birth experience, which may or may not equate with her expectations. Loving and nurturing the newborn is considered to be an inherent part of the woman's physical, emotional and psychological capacity. Western culture perpetuates the image of the woman who copes admirably with labour and birth and is unruffled by the demands of parenthood (Jebali 1993). Unfortunately this serves to invoke feelings of guilt and inadequacy and may suppress attempts to seek help for symptoms of postnatal depression. Emotions are often portrayed as tearfulness and mood swings during the first week after delivery, whilst emotional and psychological adjustment takes place. This is commonly referred to as the 'maternity blues'. The maternity blues is considered by most to be a normal sequel of childbirth. The incidence is approximately 50–80%.

It is suggested that 20% of women who suffer from maternity blues are at greater risk of developing postnatal depression (Zachary et al 1995). Postnatal depression is characterised as mental ill health and reduces the ability to think clearly and coherently. It interferes with the ability to recognise emotions of anger, fear, joy and grief and express them appropriately. Ultimately it removes the ability to cope with stress, tension and anxiety (see Box 9.1). Postnatal depression should be distinguished from postpartum psychosis, which is a more severe condition and relatively rare, with an incidence of 0.1 to 0.2%. The symptoms include hallucinations and thoughts of self-harm. Immediate psychiatric assessment is required. Postnatal depression is reported to affect 10–15% of all women who have delivered and occurs during the early postpartum weeks (O'Haro 1997). Generally episodes of postnatal depression begin within 2 to 4 weeks after the birth and can last for 2 to 6 months, but usually resolve within 1 year (Gorodetsky, Trapnell & Hamilton 1992). A large proportion of postnatal depression, however, is undetected (Seeley, Murray & Cooper 1996), with over half the cases unrecognised (Kumar 1994).

There were five reported deaths during pregnancy from suicide between 1994 and 1996, each of which involved a degree of depressive symptoms. Of the 18 deaths from suicide occurring within 1 year of delivery, there was a depressive illness noted in 11 cases as a significant predisposing factor. In many cases there were warnings which seemed to have been undetected (DOH 1998a). The confidential enquiries into maternal deaths stated that most of the women who died had repeated contact with professionals within the maternity services and as such there may have been opportunities for prevention which were lost (DOH 1998a). The government proposes to adopt a national strategy for mental health by setting a target to reduce deaths from suicide and undetermined injury by 17% by the year 2010 (Secretary of State for Health 1998). A draft national contract has set measures to meet the target by using a multiagency approach. Strategies to meet the target include tackling social exclusion, reducing isolation by a transport policy and increasing public awareness.

Attempts to categorise the signs and symptoms of postnatal depression (Box 9.1) into a diagnosable labelled illness are contended by Paradice (1995), who suggests that the signs and symptoms described can be considered a normal response to the demands of becoming a mother. Similarly, Green (1998) suggests that women experience mood changes

Reflection points

- Reflect on cases where the signs detailed in Box 9.1 may have been apparent. Which cultural factors may present as a smokescreen for the identification of postnatal illness risk factors?

- How effective are the screening tools currently used in your area of practice?

Box 9.1 **Signs that may alert the midwife to the possibility that a mother is depressed**

Tension and irritability may be expressed
Panic attacks may be experienced, presenting symptoms of tachycardia, hyperventilation and faintness (Cox 1986)
Exhaustion may be apparent with increasing sleep problems above and beyond the demands of the baby (Cox 1986)
Self-blame and low self-esteem (Kendall & Zealley 1993)
Unrealistic expectations of self and the baby
Acute anxiety over the well being of the baby
Frequent complaints of headaches, abdominal pains and breast tenderness with no adequate physical cause (Glazener et al 1995)

from feelings of exhilaration and elation to feelings of sorrow and despair during the postnatal period and may show no signs of clinical depression. Midwives are reminded to be mindful of careless labelling when the misery of motherhood could be misinterpreted as postnatal depression (Barclay & Lloyd 1996).

Factors which predispose to postnatal depression

Biological factors

Each culture provides its members with ways of viewing, describing and determining illness. Mental illness therefore is explained by some cultures, for example, as witchcraft, spirit possession and divine retribution – explanations commonly associated with non-Western ideas (Helman 1990). The Western perspective, however, emphasises aetiology based in the physical world and refers to psychological factors, life's stressors and biology as major aetiological factors. Midwives should be mindful of culturally defined concepts of health and illness when screening for postnatal illness and offering support and guidance to women and their families.

The sudden withdrawal of pregnancy hormones after childbirth was previously considered to be the biochemical factor that predisposed to postnatal depression. To date there is no conclusive evidence to support this (Harris 1993, Owens & Nemeroff 1994, Stowe & Nemeroff 1995). Other theories include the dysfunctional thyroid as a factor which predisposes to postnatal depression (Harris 1994). Investigation into thyroid dysfunction was primarily influenced by symptoms of hypothyroidism and postnatal depression occurring around the same time. Critics of this theory suggest that thyroid dysfunction could be secondary to immunological changes brought about by stress (Cooper & Murray 1998). The role of serotonin in the pathophysiology of postnatal depression is well documented (Owens & Nemeroff 1994). As serum tryptophan is the rate-limiting step in the synthesis of serotonin, low levels of the former may be viewed as a predictor for postnatal depression. Consistent findings of women with postnatal depression have demonstrated low levels of serum tryptophan (an essential amino acid necessary for growth) 4 to 5 days postpartum. It is also associated with the maternity blues and also found to be reduced in postnatally depressed women at their 6 month follow-up visits (Barker, Handley & Waldron 1981, Handley et al 1980). The theory was partly discredited when treatment with tryptophan failed to prevent the development of the maternity blues indicating that it has no influence, or that there is a possible interference in its uptake mechanism (Harris 1980).

Psychosocial factors

Predisposing risk factors which pose the most convincing aetiology are history of psychiatric disorder (see Box 9.2), history of postnatal depression, complications during childbirth and socioeconomic disadvantage. Studies of association between postnatal depression and advancing maternal age, parity, social class and educational ability produced ambiguous results. Consistent associations, however, are found with socioeconomic disadvantage and stressful life events. The most commonly cited factors found to increase the risk of postnatal depression include: marital conflict (Cooper & Murray 1998, Gallagher et al 1997, Gotlib et al 1991, Whiffen 1988), low levels of support from the partner (Cooper & Murray 1998, Graff, Dyck & Schallow 1991), child-related stressors including problems with feeding and sleeping (Cutrona 1983, Gotlib et al 1991), lack of social support, unemployment and poverty (Cooper et al 1996). Similar results have been found in other studies including research carried out by Beck (1998). To determine the level of the relationship between postnatal depression and the potential predictors of the disorder, Beck (1998) conducted a meta-analysis. Eight predictors were identified as having a significant association with postnatal depression. These included: prenatal depression (that is, depression which may occur during any trimester), child care stress (which involves, for example, stressful events relating to a child who cries frequently and does not feed well), life stress (characterised as positive or negative events), lack of social support (categorised as instrumental support like, for example, baby sitting and emotional support), prenatal anxiety (including apprehension and unease concerning, for example, nebulous threats), maternity blues, marital dissatisfaction and previous history of depression. The predictors were used to develop a screening tool, discussed later. The woman's relationship with her own mother has been found to influence the predisposition to postnatal depression. Murray et al (1995) found that women who experienced postnatal depression were more likely to have had a poor relationship with their mother. The results, however, have been questioned as no association was made with controls who experienced other forms of depression. In summary it is evident that postnatal depression is an interplay of social, biological and psychological factors.

Implications for the child

The maternal and infant relationship plays an important role in infant behavioural and cognition development. The following studies highlight the negative impact that postnatal depression may have in terms of impaired cognition and emotional development.

Reflection points

- Should the midwife be concerned?
- What action should the midwife take?
- What should the midwife detail in the antenatal records?

Box 9.2 **Case study: Mrs Jones-Butler**

Mrs Jones-Butler is a 43-year-old primigravida. She has a long-standing history of manic depressive illness. This information is not disclosed during the booking interview but the midwife is aware of the history from information reported in the general practitioner's referral letter. The midwife attempts to discuss the psychiatric history on several occasions but Mrs Jones-Butler disregards enquiries made by the midwife as futile. She explains that she is perfectly well and is looking forward to starting a new life with the baby. Her husband is equally delighted about the pregnancy, which seems to have helped their marriage problems. They both view it as the beginning of the rest of their lives. Mrs Jones-Butler is 12 weeks' pregnant. She has made all the preparations for the forthcoming birth and is at present decorating the nursery.

Accumulating evidence suggests that postnatal depression is associated with disturbances in child cognition and emotional development (Murray & Cooper 1997). A Cambridge study found that infants at 18 months whose mothers had suffered from postnatal depression performed significantly less well on cognitive tasks than did infants of well mothers. The association was found to be stronger with boys (Murray 1992, et al 1996a). Long term follow up reported by Cogill et al (1986) and Sharp et al (1995) showed that the effects continued, and were still prevalent, at the age of 5 years. The children were more likely than a control group to be described as being behaviourally disturbed at school. This study, however, was representative of a socioeconomically disadvantaged population, which may have an influence on cognition ability owing to the effects of social deprivation and poverty. Murray & Sinclair (1998) identified gender as being a predisposing factor to the longevity of the effects of postnatal depression on the child. They found that boys were more likely to be emotionally affected. Evidence suggests that poor emotional adjustment and insecure attachments are prevalent features (Lyons-Ruth et al 1986, Teti et al 1995).

It is clear so far that the impaired pattern of communication between mother and infant during an episode of postnatal depression directly affects the cognitive and emotional development of the child into early infancy. It has also been suggested that this continues into later life where children have problems in forming social attachments (Murray & Stein 1991). More recently, research has shown that unresolved emotional distress in childhood is an important cause of emotional distress in adulthood (Rutter 1996). Parent programmes which encourage the development of empathy and respect improve self-esteem in children and parents. They have also been found to increase their ability to give and receive social and emotional support (Bond & Burns 1998, Stewart-Brown 1998).

The role of antenatal education in the detection of postnatal depression

Continuity of care during the antenatal, intrapartum and postnatal period enables the midwife to know and understand the woman's mood and behaviour and extreme changes are therefore easier to detect. Research trials have established that continuity of care significantly benefits both physical and psychological outcomes in the immediate postnatal period (Hodnett 1998). The partner's behaviour may also have changed and their needs for information and support should not be underestimated. Antenatal detection of postnatal depression is possible as anxiety and depression experienced during pregnancy are associated with its prevalence postnatally (Gotlib et al 1991). A study carried out by Murray et al (1996b), presents an opposing argument. This study found that neonatal factors, including irritability and poor motor control and maternity blues, were significantly related to the onset of postnatal depression, more so than predictive antenatal factors.

Antenatal education provides an appropriate opportunity to discuss postnatal depression. Without it the likelihood of women seeking help would be markedly reduced. A survey of 78 mothers with postnatal depression showed that 90% felt that something was wrong but only 12% had spoken to a health professional about their feelings, and only 32% associated their feelings with postnatal depression (Whitton 1996). Raising awareness of the nature of the disorder may alert women and their partners to the symptoms and therefore prompt them to seek help (Elliot, Sanjak & Leverton 1988, Gruen 1990, Sharp 1996). The findings from a recent research study support this assertion. Okano et al (1998) found that women who attended antenatal education and suffered from postnatal depression were more likely to receive early psychiatric referral, with a subsequent reduction in the severity of the illness, than control counterparts. It is important to educate the woman and her partner about the symptoms of depression as for many women this may be their first encounter with a depressive episode. Discussing the difference between the 'third day blues' and postnatal depression may remove some of the fear and anxiety that women may feel about the subject. Discussing the subject antenatally may encourage women to discuss symptoms postnatally without the fear of being labelled as a bad mother (Gruen 1990, Mauthner 1997). Mauthner (1997) reported findings from a research study which sought to understand postnatal depression from a mother's point of view. The results clearly identified a need for postnatal depression to be included in an appropriate manner in antenatal education. When it was included, some women from the study group felt that health professionals running the classes were reluctant to explore the subject in detail. There is a fear that discussing postnatal depression with prospective parents may cause unnecessary anxiety and predispose them to the condition (Combes & Schonveld 1992). Raising awareness during the antenatal period has many benefits. Antenatal education involving psychosocial aspects of parenting and postnatal depression may help to heighten awareness and enable the recognition of symptoms. Midwives should explore their personal fears and anxieties with regards to addressing emotive subjects and assess their knowledge about postnatal depression. This may enable an effective and appropriate facilitation of the subject.

Providing clients with contact points where continued support can be provided is invaluable. Organisations within the United Kingdom include: the Association for Postnatal Illness, Cry-sis, the National Childbirth Trust and Home Start. Unfortunately, however, it is very difficult for some women to seek help, particularly from organisations where the financial burden of receiving help rests with the woman. Ethnic groups are also disadvantaged, particularly those who speak little or no English.

Prevention strategies and the importance of debriefing

During the intrapartum period the midwife should be aware of the woman's expectations of childbirth and how this differs from the actual event. This can be used as a trigger for discussion during the debriefing session. It should be carried out by the midwife who has supported the woman throughout the delivery experience, or the doctor when appropriate. The midwife should also be available for support during these times. The timing of debriefing should be left to the discretion of the woman after discussion with the midwife. Debriefing which takes place too near to the event may be clouded by the emotion of the experience. Conversely, if the process occurs too long after the event a distortion of reality may be evident, owing to poor memory recall. Individuals have an inherent ability to recycle through the stages of the experience, placing value judgements from self and significant others on the actual experience if they are left to speculate for long periods of time. Debriefing sessions, if led appropriately, may benefit the psychological well being of the woman. Rose (1997) defines debriefing as a psychological intervention which aims to reduce psychological morbidity after a traumatic event. This criteria leaves little room for those women who do not consider their experience traumatic but feel unhappy about the nature of the experience. In the context of this chapter, debriefing is taken to mean a process whereby the midwife uses counselling skills to discuss the birth process. Debriefing provides an opportunity for the woman and her partner to explore their thoughts and feelings about the birth process. The debriefing session should involve a full discussion of the sequence of events leading up to the birth, the nature of the birth and any fears and anxieties the woman and her partner have about the birth should be addressed at this time.

The woman should be offered a further opportunity to discuss the birth details if she so desires. This should be carried out by the same practitioner. The second debriefing session may clarify thoughts and feelings previously left unresolved from the first session. Bergin & Lambert (1978) suggest that one discussion session is enough for most women. The number of sessions should be flexible, enabling women to utilise the service as the need arises. The process of debriefing enables an opportunity for women to clarify and discuss the birth process, relate the actual experience to the previously planned experience, explore if they differ and why they differ, and discuss feelings of disappointment and self-doubt. This may also be a useful time to assess the level of psychological support the woman may need and recognise postnatal depression risk factors. Holden (1994) supports this view and emphasises that discussing the birth experience can facilitate early recognition of women who are experiencing difficulties. The John Radcliffe Hospital in Oxford, England runs a programme called 'Afterthoughts', which provides an unlimited period of debriefing for women to discuss and explore their childbirth experiences. The evaluation of this service revealed that even after many years women were found to have unresolved concerns about their birth experience (Udall 1996).

The efficacy of debriefing sessions as a positive postnatal intervention has been recently tested. One hundred and fourteen postnatal primigravidas were allocated either to receive the debriefing intervention ($n = 56$), or to form the control group where no intervention was given ($n = 58$). The outcome measure used was the hospital anxiety and depression scale. Women who received the intervention were less likely than women in the control group to have high anxiety and depression scores after delivery. The researchers conclude that there are large benefits with regards to psychological well being to be gained from offering this service. They stress that all maternity units have a responsibility to provide postnatal debriefing sessions (Lavender & Walkinshaw 1998).

Discussion questions

- How important do you think debriefing is as a strategy to promote psychological well being?
- Is this process an integral part of midwifery practice?
- How could the debriefing process be formalised and recognised by stakeholders as an invaluable part of childbirth?

Screening

Studies have highlighted the inability of health professionals to diagnose postnatal depression using conventional screening methods (Holden 1989). The Edinburgh scale of depression provides a reliable basis for screening for postnatal depression. It was developed by Cox, Holden & Sagovsky (1987) as a 10-point self-reporting scale about feelings in the past week. Each item is scored 0–3. For each statement women are asked to underline one of the following four possible responses: 'as much as I could,' 'not quite so much now', 'definitely not so much now', or 'not at all.' Although it does not encourage the describing of symptoms fully it does provoke thought. Once completed, there should be an opportunity for discussion of feelings, particularly if any mother scores above the predetermined cut-off line of 12 (Holden 1991). Scores above 12 indicate negative feelings and referral for further investigation and possible diagnosis is warranted. The tool is not intended to replace clinical judgement but serves more as a form of risk assessment. It is a reliable psychometric test and in a large community study revealed a specificity of 92% and a sensitivity of 88% (Murray & Carothers 1990). Other authors report good detection rates and advocate its use (Holden 1991). Unfortunately, people who are unable to read English are very often excluded from the screening tool. Even if the tool were translated into other languages it is argued that the questionnaire would present lower scores for non-Western cultures and produce false negative results. Questionnaires designed for one culture are not necessarily valid in another (Hearn et al 1998). Helman (1990) suggests that a problem encountered when making a psychiatric diagnosis cross-culturally is somatisation. This is a cultural expression of psychological disorders into a language of signs, behaviour and physical symptoms, which is not represented in the Edinburgh scale of depression. People in non-Western cultures are more likely to complain of pain than depression and would frequently deny feeling depressed if asked. It is suggested that somatisation is more common among the poorer social groups, whereas middle class professional groups from non-Western cultures view depression as a psychological problem (Kleinman & Kleinman 1985). Beck (1998) developed a postpartum depression predictor inventory (PDPI), which after meta-analysis revealed significant predictors of postpartum depression. Unlike the Edinburgh postnatal depression scale the PDPI is not designed as a self-report questionnaire nor an intended formal instrument with tested psychometric properties. It is designed to be used during prenatal visits as a part of routine care. The tool should form part of a discussion and encourage dialogue about issues relating to predictive values including prenatal depression, prenatal anxiety, previous history of depression, lack of social support, marital dissatisfaction and life stresses. Two questions are designed for postnatal use and include child care stress and maternity blues. Literacy skills would not be necessary for the completion of the tool and there is obvious room for dialogue. Health professionals are required to use their skills to elicit information based on the questions on the tool. However, 'yes' and 'no' answers are all that is required for completion. As there is no specified score which would depict high risk cases, identification would be purely based on the information received from the discussion. Although the tool has many favourable properties, psychometric testing to determine specificity and sensitivity of the instrument is needed, for reliable detection (Beck 1998).

The Edinburgh scale of depression at present is a more reliable indicator of postnatal depression.

Treatment

Treatment based on psychological methods

Counselling by appropriately trained personnel can have a profound effect on the curtailment of the disorder and is very often the treatment of choice. A research study found that women who received nine visits over 13 weeks from health visitors trained in non-directive counselling showed improvement in their overall mood, more so than women in the control group who received conventional primary care (Holden 1989). Similar results have been noted in other studies (Cooper & Murray 1997, Wickberg & Hwang 1996). The role of the midwife in the treatment of postnatal depression is underestimated. Disturbances in the mother–child relationship begin very early in the postpartum period, during which time the midwife is the health professional with the most contact. Indeed psychosocial factors which predispose to postnatal depression may be detected early in the antenatal period. The midwife's individualised approach and the close contact that is established throughout this time may enhance detection rates. The government green paper, *Supporting families* (DOH 1998b), clearly identifies midwives and health visitors as having a role in assessing the susceptibility to postnatal depression by observing the social circumstances, family interactions and the levels of social support. A pilot scheme run by health visitors in London sought to identify tension states within the home which may influence the incidence of postnatal depression. They involved themselves in supporting women and their partners in identified areas of conflict where problems with relationships were leading to problems with parenting. Health visitors were able to explore and discuss issues to help alleviate further potential problems (Young 1998). This type of support is valuable and midwives could certainly utilise information about the resolution of conflict as a part of antenatal education. Sessions on parenting skills could include the impact of the neonate on dynamics of home life and the changing roles of parents. Commissioners and providers of maternity care should direct time and resources to this important aspect of support. It is suggested that a specialist health professional is allocated on a sessional basis for managing perinatal health. Part of this role would include liaising with maternity, community and mental health services in order to ensure continuity of recognised cases of mental illness. Contact and continuity would continue throughout the antenatal, postpartum and infant life of the family. This approach would ensure the support of appropriate professional groups and improve communication channels between them (DOH 1998b).

Support and continuity that the midwife provides continues well into the postnatal period. Detection of high risk cases, and continued support and planning, together with non-directive counselling, is a natural progression of the midwife's work with women who are postnatally depressed. The importance of early detection cannot be overemphasised, with reported findings of early detection leading to curtailment of the disease. Careful deliberate introduction of the health visitor in preparation for more extensive counselling will enhance the recovery process. A multidisciplinary approach is most certainly the better option for treatment utilising the expertise of all appropriate professional disciplines.

Drug treatment

Drug treatment can possibly produce antidepressant effects but does not in its entirety address the psychosocial factors which predispose to the aetiology of the illness. Progesterone treatment has been advocated as a drug of choice (Dalton 1985), but warrants further evaluation with regards to efficacy. More recently, however, oestrogen was found to be useful in providing antidepressive effects among a group of woman receiving the drug, more so than those who received a placebo (Gregoire et al 1996). A recent study observed the efficacy of the drug fluoxetine in comparison to the counselling approach as a treatment for postnatal depression. Both the drug and psychological treatment showed a significant antidepressant effect. The drug treatment, however, was not shown to be superior to the psychological treatment in terms of success (Appleby et al 1997). Psychological therapy in terms of counselling would appear to be therapeutic in addressing real life issues, which are often the root of the problem. For this approach to be successful, however, trained skilled counsellors are essential.

Women who are given drug therapy for the relief of postnatal depression would certainly benefit from a multidisciplinary approach to care.

Rape-related post-traumatic stress disorder – the long term sequelae for survivors of rape and sexual assault and its impact on pregnancy and childbirth

During my experience of counselling survivors of rape, the magnitude of long term trauma in survivors of rape experience has heightened my awareness of the profound effect the childbirth experience may have on areas of resolved or unresolved conflict. The high incidence of female rape infers that there is a strong possibility that survivors, at some stage in their lives, will experience childbirth. Although this is purely conjecture, and there is a dearth of research-based evidence to validate this claim, Holz (1994) estimates that approximately 30% of all women have experienced some form of sexual abuse in childhood or adolescence. This may result in long term sequelae for the survivor and present as post-traumatic stress disorder (PTSD). Flashbacks, commonly associated with the disorder, may be triggered during pregnancy and childbirth owing to the intrusive nature of midwifery and obstetric practice (see Box 9.3). This may add to the violated and depressive feelings of the survivor, whose trauma of the event has continued. The birth experience may therefore become an added trauma. Survivors of sexual abuse have described childbirth as a repetition of the rape (Christensen 1992, Kitzinger 1992). It is virtually impossible to anticipate all the effects of rape-related post-traumatic stress disorder (RRPTSD), but increased awareness and sensitivity during midwifery practice may help to reduce the severity of the symptoms during the antenatal, intrapartum and postpartum period where signs of postnatal depression may be evident. To appreciate fully the depth of the disorder, it is useful to clarify issues relating to rape.

Historical perspective – an overview

Rape and sexual assaults may include both verbal and physical attacks ranging from being 'touched up' or 'chatted up' to being brutally sexually assaulted with objects. The meanings of 'sexual assault' and the sexuality of women have changed significantly since the colonial period. At that time women were valued for their sexual purity and were viewed as the centre of the family. Sexual intercourse was acceptable only within marriage for the purpose of procreation. If a women engaged in sex outside marriage, even against her will, she was considered a fallen woman and was often blamed for her own victimisation. The behaviour of settlers in English colonies was influenced strongly by the church, which prescribed the behaviour of its congregation. Towards the end of the eighteenth century, however, sexual meanings began to change. Sex was no longer tied solely to reproduction. Courtship became more favourable. The decline in church and state regulations influenced individual control and the constraint on non-marital sex was reduced. As women from the countryside entered paid employment during the nineteenth century, patriarchal controls over women's time, behaviour and sexuality weakened further. With increased freedom came increased vulnerability. In addition to oppressing women, rape served as a method of racial control. The sexual assault of minority women maintained the supremacy of white men. The experience of the black female victim was virtually ignored. In the postreconstruction South USA, white men perpetuated the myth of the black man as sexually uncontrollable as a means of violating black men and controlling white women (D'Emilio 1992).

With the feminist movement of the 1960s rape was identified as a mechanism for maintaining male control and domination and a violent means of enforcing fear in women and reinforcing their subordination to men. The crime of rape, historically believed to have a sexual imperative, often seemed to place the burden of proof on the victim to demonstrate that she didn't deserve to be assaulted. Adulterous women, prostitutes and wives were considered 'rape proof'. Legal rights of women changed with the social changes in attitudes toward women. For example, the economic and political rights of women helped assert women's independent status. Owning their own property meant that women could seek redress for any injuries inflicted upon them rather than relying on the men in their lives. It still, however, remains increasingly difficult for women who are the survivors of 'date rape' and women who have been raped by their husbands to prove that the rape took place. People are more likely to define rape as forced intercourse between strangers and trivialise the consequences of rape when it occurs between acquaintances, during date rape and within marriages (Ward 1995). A survey carried out in North London, England assessed the prevalence of date rape and found that 9% of women had been raped and 25% touched sexually in a way they did not want to be touched. No more than five dates had taken place prior to the assault. They were not reported to the police. The main reasons given for non-reporting were 'embarrassment', 'fear of not being believed', and 'that it would not be taken seriously given that I knew the man' (Mooney 1994).

Myths and stereotypes

In addition to the outcome of the rape itself, other variables may moderate the seriousness of the victim's psychological response. Commonly held myths influence the definition of rape, the behaviour of the survivor and her significant others. Myths about rapists, which include dirty old men in plastic coats and lunatics in dark alleys, protect certain groups of people and encourage a false sense of security (Mooney 1994). It is important to remember that all social classes, all age groups and all races are capable of rape. Another strongly held idea is that the rapist is weak willed and unable to control his own sexual urges; therefore he is forced to rape. This commonly held idea is designed to do two things: first to make women responsible for rapes committed against them, and secondly to make sure that women do not deny men access to their bodies when they are sexually aroused because if they do they are forced to go out and rape. Commonly held myths about the victims include the idea that only certain types of women are raped – for example, those who stay out late at night alone, and those who dress in a way which is perceived to be provocative. Preconceptions that women have about rape prior to being raped will affect the way they view themselves. It also influences to a certain extent the amount of guilt and psychological trauma they may inflict upon themselves. It is suggested that friends, lovers, husbands, doctors, nurses and midwives often project their own version of events on to the survivor's version. This is often distorted either to fit their own theories or to protect themselves from reality. The consequences leave women denied of their experience (London Rape Crisis Centre (LRCC) 1988). It is evident then that myths and ideas about rape play a powerful part in defining rape. Health professionals must examine their own ideas about rape, the perpetrator and the survivor before they can give unbiased support to the survivor.

Factors which increase the likelihood of post-traumatic stress disorder

The attitudes and behaviours that the survivor exhibits during the course of the assault can influence the severity of the psychological consequence. More specifically, women who resist rape with physical force may be less likely to suffer from self-blame or criticism (Ward 1995) (see Fig. 9.1, p. 190).

Resistance of rape can be viewed as being positive, but when considering the viability of various resistance strategies a clear assessment of the severity of the consequences of each strategy is essential. This may involve: the severity of psychological trauma from a completed rape, the impact of a survivor's actions during the assault on her subsequent self-esteem, the probable effect of various strategies in avoiding the completion of the rape, and the relative risk of physical injury. Whichever resistance strategy the woman uses during the rape, it will be open to critical challenge and judgement by herself and others. In an attempt to assess the efficacy of resistance strategies, Ullman (1992) presented findings which put the burden of responsibility on the woman for reducing the severity of the rape. Ullman (1992) investigated the effects of two types of physical resistance: forceful fighting and screaming versus pleading, begging and reasoning. Forceful fighting and screaming were found to reduce the severity of sexual abuse, without increasing the level of physical injury. This was found to be the most effective in avoiding rape. The researcher suggests that women do not realise the ineffectiveness of pleading, begging and reasoning with the offender. If some rapists are seeking to feel powerful in their control of a weaker person, pleading may reward the rapist's behaviour. However, Ullman emphasises that, although the study showed advantages of forceful fighting, women should not be blamed if they are unable to use this resistance strategy.

Many women experience guilt feelings about being raped and think critically about what they could have done to avoid or stop it. Friends and family may add to guilt feelings by asking, 'Why didn't you ...'? Some women feel powerless to make decisions. Physical repulsion is commonly experienced.

Not being believed

The acceptance of false memory syndrome has relieved some people of their guilt. It is described as the ideal gift for the perpetrator, but has created another problem for the survivor. The fear of not being believed reduces the likelihood of disclosure and subsequent healing; it also adds to the depth of trauma and negatively influences the recovery process. This syndrome denies survivors their experiences by suggesting that the whole experience was dreamed up, thus absolving the perpetrator of any distasteful behaviour (Mezey 1994).

Long term sequelae

Pre-existing factors, including psychological problems and chronic life stressors, influence the recovery process (Burgess 1995, Mynatt & Allgeier 1990).

Examination fears

The consequences of rape on women's health should not be underestimated. For some survivors the fear of being examined means that they avoid attendance for cervical screening or antenatal care. The medical encounter, which combines nakedness, touching, intrusion, pain or discomfort and powerlessness or depersonalisation, often leaves women feeling humiliated, dirty and violated. Kitzinger (1990) suggests that it can reproduce the dynamics of sexual violence (see Box 9.3). A survey which explored the perceptions of survivors of sexual abuse has shown that 65–67% believed that the abuse had a long term defective effect on their lives, producing or adding to low self-esteem and problems with starting or maintaining a loving relationship (Baker & Duncan 1985). Health professionals may be unaware of the abuse, but can remain sensitive to the woman's needs, acknowledge non-verbal behaviour and attempt to promote a safe

Box 9.3 **Pregnancy and childbirth: survivors' perceptions of trauma related to midwife procedures**

Perceptions of procedure:
Exposure of body parts: abdominal palpation, vaginal examination, lithotomy position
Position of inferiority: lying on the couch/bed during procedures
Being touched and pressed: abdominal palpation, vaginal examination, perineal repair
Invasion of body space: listening to the fetal heart with a pinnard stethoscope
Force and manipulation: forceps, ventouse delivery, management of a shoulder dystocia
Genital pain and trauma: tears, episiotomy, bruising, postpartum bleeding

Actions of the practitioner which may be perceived as trauma triggers:
Rubbing hands together to make them warm prior to abdominal palpation
Facial expression of intrigue, during vaginal examination, verbalising intrigue as in mm, ahh, etc.
Careful, deliberate parting the labia majora prior to inserting fingers for vaginal examination
Holding the entonox mouthpiece or mask on to the woman's face
Opening the woman's legs and observing her sanitary towel
Administering a pain-relieving suppository

environment for the woman who may experience a problem during examination. It may be useful to reflect on the number and nature of examinations performed on a woman during pregnancy, labour and the postnatal period, and consider the consequences of what is perceived to be unnecessary and intrusive behaviour (see Box 9.3).

Post-traumatic stress disorder

A reaction to being exposed to an event or sequence of events which is beyond normal human experience can be referred to as post-traumatic stress disorder. Any event which leaves the individual psychologically traumatised provides a broader scope for the definition. Experiences may include: rape, sexual assault, domestic violence, child abuse, accidents, natural disasters and childbirth. Reber (1985) defines PTSD as a psychological disorder associated with serious traumatic events. Adult survivors carry the legacy of physical, emotional and spiritual trauma for many years into their adult lives. This may be presented in different forms of psychiatric and somatic problems. PTSD is further described as 'maladaptive symptoms arising from rape and other forms of sexual abuse' (Ward 1995 p. 118). In an attempt to demonstrate the process of PTSD

Figure 9.1
Stress and coping framework (from Ward 1995, with permission of Sage)

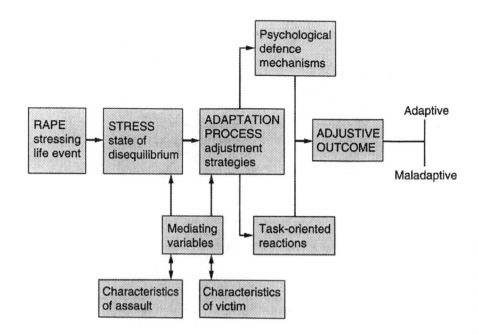

and the influences associated with its severity Ward (1995) presented a conceptual framework of stress and coping (Fig. 9.1). The framework acknowledges the different responses to crisis and infers the relative unpredictability involved in the adaptive process to the stressor. Unpredictability is largely influenced by: the nature of the rape, resistance strategies used during the rape, the responses of friends, family and health practitioners and the cultural background of the survivor, which influences her personal ideas and beliefs about rape. Mediating variables positively or negatively influence the severity of the response to trauma; family rape and date rape studies have presented evidence of differential response (Ward 1995).

Burgess (1995) describes four diagnostic criteria of rape-related PTSD:

- The stressor is of such a magnitude that it evokes distinguishable symptoms.
- The trauma is re-experienced, including flashbacks.
- Reduction of personal involvement with the environment or detachment from the reality of living (this may affect family and social relations where the survivor becomes abstract to her own life).
- Exhibition of two symptoms from the following list: exaggerated startle response or hyperalertness, disturbance in sleep pattern, guilt about surviving or behaviour displayed during the rape, impairment of memory and/or power of concentration, avoidance of activities that arouse recollection,

and increased symptoms to the event that symbolise or resemble the event (this may cause vaginismus when vaginal examination is attempted during labour, reduction or absence of antenatal clinic appointments, avoidance of cervical smears and self breast examination).

The most common problem experienced is depression, often misdiagnosed as bipolar disease. Other common behaviours and problems include: inability to trust and form intimate relationships, sexual dysfunction, addictive behaviours, self-destructive tendencies, poor self-esteem, phobias and multiple somatic complaints (Holz 1994). Parratt (1994) sought to identify what experiences women who are survivors of incest have during childbirth. Interview data indicated that memories of abuse may return during labour and delivery. Trauma as a result of provoked memories vary in depth and nature and may be influenced by: the age the sexual abuse began, whether there were multiple perpetrators, if the survivor was believed and if sexual intercourse took place (Morrow 1991). Lack of support and treatment increases the chances of long term effects and the prevalence of PTSD (Lowery 1987).

Trauma is perceived in different ways. Box 9.3 lists normal procedural practices for the midwife, which may be viewed as traumatic by the woman suffering from rape-related PTSD. If the woman is already vulnerable owing to previous traumatic events, then pregnancy and childbirth may cause her to relive the experience. Symptoms of the disorder may be prevalent soon after the trauma or may not be evident until many years later. It is not unusual for symptoms to become apparent during times of stress and further trauma. Symptoms of PTSD include (Burgess & Holmstrom 1974):

- lack of concentration
- feelings of depression and isolation
- inability to trust others
- hypervigilence
- feelings of helplessness
- feelings of fear
- experiencing flashbacks by triggers associated with the trauma
- avoidance of known triggers which may cause flashbacks
- dreams about the event
- mood swings and irritability
- embarrassment and shame
- change in eating patterns, loss of appetite
- lack of confidence and low self-esteem
- change in sleep patterns
- feelings of being dirty
- muscular tension, gastrointestinal irritability.

Flashbacks

Symptoms of flashbacks of trauma can be quite profound. A flashback in this situation is characterised as the traumatic event intruding into everyday life. The event seems once again real and vivid for the woman, who may lose her sense of what is reality and what is memory. The feeling that the abuse is happening again may, therefore, become apparent. During the flashback the woman may experience sensory and motor reenactments, or may faint during the experience. Recollection of what happened during the flashback is rare. Consideration of the events perceived as traumatic during childbirth may enable the midwife to have a deeper understanding of strategies which may be utilised to avoid such triggers (see Box 9.3).

Avoidance strategies

Avoidance strategies in relation to maternity care include: refusal to have procedures considered to be invasive take place, guarding or maintaining modesty excessively, an inability to explain symptoms or indeed remember (as many trauma survivors forget in order to survive). Avoidance strategies also include the survivor 'switching off' during a stressful event. This is classically illustrated as disassociation and may be apparent during childbirth. No emotion may be expressed. The midwife may perceive this as disinterest, but for the woman this may mean survival. Due to the need to avoid situations and circumstances, from an inability to work through feelings experienced following a traumatic event, the survivor is left with the trauma controlling her life. This will inevitably lead to depression.

In conclusion, pregnancy and childbirth may invoke feelings of trauma that are very often hidden by the abused woman. However, it is not somebody else's problem. Also, before midwives are able to support women who have been raped or sexuality assaulted they must examine their own myths and ideas about rape.

The midwife's role – developing a therapeutic relationship

It is difficult for the midwife to recognise that a woman is suffering from rape-related PTSD. The criteria listed by Burgess & Holmstrom (1974) are a useful indicator, but by no means exhaustive. Somatisation may be apparent in people of other cultures and their expression of symptoms may differ. Developing a close relationship with the client may render deviations from the normal recognisable, however. The symptoms of the disorder previously described are graphic vivid accounts, the feelings of which continue to control people's lives. Preparation for childbirth may invoke feelings of fear and anxiety. A relationship with the woman that is based on trust, empathy, genuineness, respect and confidentiality may build therapeutic links and nurture painful feelings. The following principles may support the basic requirements of a therapeutic relationship. Safety is a fundamental aspect of this approach. Without foundations of safety, counselling skills will not be mutually regarded (see Ch. 4).

Points for guidance include the following.

- Continuity of care is essential to enable the development of a therapeutic relationship.
- Good listening skills are important, as cries for help may be deliberately hidden.
- Antenatal classes are not usually used as therapeutic groups. Clients who discuss or wish to explore painful events repeatedly, regardless of the subject, may need further support and help. Recognising when to refer a client for specialist support is important.
- Preparation for labour and teaching parenting skills may be more appropriate on a one to one basis.
- In the event of a flashback stand close by, and make the area safe. After the flashback offer open dialogue. Forced questioning removes the woman's control.
- Postdelivery debriefing is essential, but should not be forced. An open door policy may be offered.
- It is important to recognise when a helping relationship becomes a counselling relationship.

Reflection points

- Consider actions that you have taken or observed which have the potential to produce a flashback response.
- Think about the relationship you have with clients and boundaries, which may promote, or prevent disclosure of problems associated with rape-related post-traumatic stress disorder.
- Consider helping strategies you would use if exposed to invoked feelings of trauma.

Summary

- Postnatal depression is reported to affect 10–15% of all women who have delivered and occurs during the early postpartum weeks.
- The most commonly cited factors found to increase the risk of postnatal depression include: marital conflict, low levels of support from the partner, child-related stressors including problems with feeding and sleeping, lack of social support, unemployment and poverty.
- There is little evidence to support a biological aetiology, but antenatal, personal and social factors are relevant.
- Postnatal depression is associated with disturbances in child cognition and emotional development. Unresolved emotional distress in childhood is an important cause of emotional distress in adulthood.

- Antenatal education provides an appropriate opportunity to discuss postnatal depression. Raising awareness of the nature of the disorder can help women and their partners to be alert to the symptoms and therefore prompt them to seek help.
- Continuity of care during the antenatal, intrapartum and postnatal period enables the midwife to know and understand the woman's mood and behaviour and extreme changes are therefore easier to detect.
- Midwives should explore their personal fears and anxieties with regards to addressing emotive subjects and assess their knowledge about postnatal depression. This may enable the effective and appropriate facilitation of the subject.
- Debriefing sessions, if led appropriately, may benefit the psychological well being of the woman. All maternity units have a responsibility to provide postnatal debriefing sessions. Providers of maternity services should be allocated sufficient resources to offer debriefing to all users as an integral part of service provision.
- The Edinburgh scale of depression provides a reliable basis for screening for postnatal depression. The tool is not intended to replace clinical judgement but serves more as a form of risk assessment. A problem may be encountered when making a psychiatric diagnosis cross-culturally using the Edinburgh scale of depression as it may produce false negative results.
- Counselling has been found to be an effective intervention and can be delivered by midwives and health visitors.
- Drug treatment can possibly produce antidepressant effects but does not in its entirety address the psychosocial factors which predispose to the aetiology of the illness.
- Rape myths influence the perceptions of and responses to survivors of rape. As health professionals it is important to examine, reflect upon, and clarify our own ideas and myths about rape in order to be objective participants in the care of women who disclose abuse. The myths held by members of society can influence not only how one reacts to another who has been raped but also how the survivor of rape will feel about her own self-worth.
- The attitudes and behaviours that the survivors exhibit during the course of the assault can influence the severity of the psychological consequences. More specifically, women who resist rape with physical force may be less likely to suffer from self blame or criticism.
- A reaction to being exposed to an event or sequence of events which is beyond normal human experience can be referred to as post-traumatic stress disorder.

- Events in pregnancy and childbirth which may invoke feelings of trauma are very often hidden by the abused woman. In particular, examinations which are intrusive in nature should be questioned with regards to frequency and rationale.
- Flashbacks, commonly associated with the disorder, may be triggered during pregnancy and childbirth, owing to the intrusive nature of midwifery and obstetric practice.
- Denial and refashioning the experience to make it seem less serious is a common approach to dealing with the problems. Encouraging the woman to get over the experience, being dismissive or informing her that it isn't all that bad can only serve to traumatise her further.
- It is difficult for the midwife to recognise that a woman is suffering from rape-related PTSD. Developing a close relationship with the client renders deviations from the normal recognisable to the midwife.

References

Appleby L, Warner R, Whitton A, Faragher B 1997 A controlled study: fluoxetine and cognitive-behavioural counselling in the treatment of postnatal depression. British Medical Journal 314:932–936

Baker A, Duncan S 1985 Child sexual abuse: a study of prevalence in Great Britain. Child Abuse and Neglect 9:457–467

Barclay L, Lloyd B 1996 The misery of motherhood: alternative approaches to maternal distress. Midwifery 12:136–139

Barker J M, Handley S L, Waldron G 1981 Seasonal variations in plasma tryptophan in parturient women. Progress in Neuropsychopharmacology 5:515–518

Beck C T 1998 A check list to identify women at risk for developing postpartum depression. Journal of Obstetric, Gynaecological and Neonatal Nursing 27(1):39–46

Bergin A E, Lambert M J 1978 The evaluation of therapeutic outcomes. In: Garfield S L, Bergin A E (eds) Handbook of psychotherapy and behaviour change. John Wiley, New York, pp 139–189

Bond L, Burns C 1998 Investing in parents' development as an investment in primary prevention. Journal of Mental Health (7)5:493–503

Burgess A 1995 Rape trauma syndrome. In: Searles P, Berger R (eds) Rape and society, readings on the problem of sexual assault. Westview Press, Boulder CO, p 102

Burgess A W, Holmstrom L L 1974 Rape trauma syndrome. American Journal of Psychiatry 131:981–986

Christensen M 1992 Birth rape. Midwifery Today 22(34):17–20

Cogill S, Caplan H, Alexandra H, Robson K, Kumar R 1986 Impact of postnatal depression on cognitive development of young children. British Medical Journal 292:1165–1167

Combes G, Schonveld A 1992 Life will never be the same again: a review of antenatal and postnatal health education. Health Education Authority, London

Cooper P J, Murray L 1997 The impact of psychological treatments of postpartum depression on maternal mood and infant development. In: Murray L, Cooper P J (eds) Postpartum depression and child development. Guilford, New York, pp 201–220

Cooper P J, Murray L 1998 Postnatal depression. British Medical Journal 316(7148):1884–1886

Cooper P J, Murray L, Hooper R, West A 1996 The development and validation of a predictive index for postpartum depression. Psychological Medicine 26:627–634

Cox J L 1986 Postnatal depression – a guide for health professionals. Churchill Livingstone, New York

Cox J L, Holden J M, Sagovsky R 1987 Detection of postnatal depression. Development of the 10-item Edinburgh Postnatal Depression Scale. British Journal of Psychiatry 150:782–786

Cutrona C E 1983 Causal attributions of perinatal depression. Journal of Abnormal Psychology 92:161–172

Dalton K 1985 Progesterone prophylaxis used sucessfully in postnatal depression. Practitioner:229–508

Department of Health (DOH) 1998a Why mothers die – report on the confidential enquiries into maternal deaths in the United Kingdom 1994–1996. The Stationery Office, London

Department of Health (DOH) 1998b Supporting families. The Stationery Office, London

Elliot S A, Sanjak M, Leverton T 1988 Parent groups in pregnancy: a preventive intervention for postnatal depression? In: Gottlieb B H (ed) Marshalling social support. Formats, processes and effects. Sage, Beverley Hills CA, pp 78–90

D'Emilio J 1992 A feminist redefinition of rape and sexual assault. Historical foundations for change. Journal of Interpersonal Violence 9(4):39–42

Gallagher R, Steven E, Ritter C, Ritter S, Lavin J 1997 Marriage, intimate support and depression during pregnancy. Journal of Health Psychology 2(4):457–469

Glazener C M A, Abdalla M I, Stroud P, Naji S A, Templeton A A, Russell I T 1995 Postnatal maternal morbidity: extent, cause, prevention, treatment. British Journal of Obstetrics and Gynaecology 102:282–287

Gorodetsky G M, Trapnell R H, Hamilton J A 1992 Major postpartum depression. In: Hamilton J A, Harberger P N (eds) Postpartum psychiatric illness: a picture puzzle. University of Pennsylvania Press, Philadelphia

Gotlib I, Whiffen V E, Wallace P, Mount J H 1991 A prospective investigation of postpartum depression: factors involved in onset and recovery. Journal of Abnormal Psychology 100:122–132

Graff L A, Dyck D G, Schallow J R 1991 Predicting postpartum depressive symptoms: a structural modelling analysis. Perceptual and Motor Skills 73:1137–1138

Green J M 1998 Postnatal depression or perinatal dysphoria? Findings from a longitudinal community based study using the Edinburgh postnatal depression scale. Journal of Reproductive and Infant Psychology 16(2):143–155

Gregoire A J P, Kumar R, Everitt B, Henderson A F, Studd J W W 1996 Transdermal oestrogen for treatment of severe postnatal depression. Lancet 347:930–933

Gruen D S 1990 Postpartum depression: a debilitating yet often unassessed problem. Health and Social Work 15:261–270

Handley S L, Dunn T L, Waldron G et al 1980 Trytophan, cortisol and puerperal mood. British Journal of Psychiatry 136:498–508

Harris B 1980 Prospective trial of L-tryptophan in maternity blues. British Journal of Psychiatry 137:233–235

Harris B 1993 A hormonal component to postnatal depression. British Journal of Psychiatry 163:403–405

Harris B 1994 Biological and hormonal aspects of postpartum depressed mood. British Journal of Psychiatry 164:288–292

Hearn G, Iliff A, Jones I et al 1998 Postnatal depression in the community. British Journal of General Practice 48:1064–1066

Helman C G 1990 Culture, health and illness. Butterworth-Heinemann, Oxford

Hodnett E 1998 Support from caregivers during childbirth. In: Cochrane database of systematic reviews, issue 2. Update Software, Oxford

Holden J 1989 Counselling in a general practice setting: a controlled study of health visitor intervention in the treatment of postnatal depression. British Medical Journal 298:223–236

Holden J M 1991 Postnatal depression: its nature, effects and identification using the Edinburgh depression scale. Birth 18:211–221

Holden J M 1994 Can non-psychotic depression be prevented? In: Cox J, Holden J (eds) Perinatal psychiatry: use and misuse of the Edinburgh Postnatal Depression scale. Gaskell, London, pp 78–80

Holz K 1994 A practical approach to clients who are survivors of childhood sexual abuse. Journal of Nurse-Midwifery 39(1):13–18

Jebali C A 1993 A feminist perspective on postnatal depression. Health Visitor 66(2):59–60

Kendall R, Zealley A 1993 Companion to psychiatric studies, vol 5. Churchill Livingstone, New York

Kitzinger J 1990 Recalling the pain. Nursing Times 86(3) (January):20–22

Kitzinger J 1992 Counteracting, not reenacting, the violation of women's bodies: the challenge for perinatal care givers. Birth 19(4):219–220

Kleinman A, Kleinman J 1985 Somatization. In: Kleinman A, Good B (eds) Culture and depression. University of California Press, Berkeley CA, pp 429–490

Kumar R C 1994 Postnatal depression. Maternal and Child Health 19:354–358

Lavender T, Walkinshaw S 1998 Can midwives reduce postpartum psychological morbidity? A randomized trial. Birth 25 (4 December):215–218

London Rape Crisis Centre (LRCC) 1988 Sexual violence the reality for women. LRCC, London

Lowery M 1987 Adult survivors of childhood incest. Journal of Psychosocial Nursing and Mental Health Services 24(1)

Lyons-Ruth K, Zoll D, Connell D, Grunebaum H U 1986 The depressed mother and her one year old infant: environment, interaction and attachment and infant development. In: Tronick E Z, Field T (eds) Maternal depression and infant disturbance. New directions for child development. Jossey-Bass, San Francisco CA, p 34

Mauthner N S 1997 Postnatal depression: how can midwives help? Midwifery 13(4):163–171

Mezey G 1994 Is false memory syndrome the real fiction? (press release). Accuracy About Abuse.

Mooney J 1994 The hidden figure: domestic violence in North London. Islington County Council, London

Morrow K 1991 Attributions of female adolescent incest victims regarding their molestation. Child Abuse and Neglect 14(4):126–130

Murray D, Cox D, Chapman G, Jones P 1995 Childbirth: life event or start of long term difficulty? Further data from the Stoke on Trent controlled study of postnatal depression. British Journal of Psychiatry 166(5):595–600

Murray L 1992 The impact of postnatal depression on child development. Journal of Child Psychology and Psychiatry 33:543–561

Murray L, Carothers A D 1990 The validation of the Edinburgh postnatal depression scale on a community sample. British Journal of Psychiatry 157:288–290

Murray L, Cooper P J 1997 Effects of postnatal depression on infant development. Archives of Disease in Childhood 77:99–101

Murray L, Sinclair D 1998 Effects of postnatal depression on children's adjustment to school. British Journal of Psychiatry 172:58–63

Murray L, Stein A 1991 The effects of postnatal depression on mother-infant relations and infant development. In: Woodhead M, Carr R, Light P (eds) Becoming a person. Routledge, London, pp 65–71

Murray L, Fiori-Cowley A, Hooper R, Cooper P J 1996a The impact of postnatal depression and associated adversity on early mother-infant interactions and later infant outcome. Child Development 67:2512–2526

Murray L, Stanley C, Hooper R, King F, Fiori-Cowley A 1996b The role of infant factors in postnatal depression and mother–infant interactions. Developmental Medicine and Child Neurology 38:109–119

Mynatt C R, Allgeier E R 1990 Risk factors, self attributions and adjustment problems among victims of sexual coercion. Journal of Applied Social Psychology 20:92–101

O'Haro M W 1997 The nature of postpartum depressive disorders. In: Murray L, Cooper P J (eds) Postpartum depression and child development. Guilford, New York, pp 3–31

Okano T, Nagata S, Hasegaara M et al 1998 Effectiveness of antenatal education about postnatal depression: a comparison of two groups of Japanese mothers. Journal of Mental Health 7(2):191–198

Owens M J, Nemeroff C B 1994 The role of serotonin in the pathophysiology of depression: focus on the serotonin transporter. Clinical Chemistry 40:288–295

Paradice K 1995 Postnatal depression: a normal response to motherhood? British Journal of Midwifery 3(12) (December):632–635

Parratt J 1994 The experience of childbirth for survivors of incest. Midwifery 10:26–39

Prescott-Clarke P, Primatesta P (eds) 1997 Health survey for England 1995: findings of a survey carried out on the behalf of the Department of Health, London. Series HS, 8(1). The Stationery Office, London

Reber A 1985 Dictionary of psychology. Penguin Books, London, p 799

Rose S 1997 Psychological debriefing: history and methods. Counselling 8:48–51

Rutter M 1996 Connections between child and adult psychopathology, European Clinical Adolescent Psychology 5(suppl) 1:4–7

Secretary of State for Health 1998 Our healthier nation, a contract for health. A consultation paper. The Stationery Office, London

Seeley S, Murray L, Cooper P J 1996 Postnatal depression: the outcome for mothers and babies of health visitor intervention. Health Visitor 69:135–138

Sharp D 1996 The prevention of postnatal depression. In: Kendrick T, Tylee A, Freeling P (eds) The prevention of mental illness in primary care. Cambridge University Press, Cambridge, pp 76–80

Sharp D, Hay D, Pawlby S, Schmucher G, Allen H, Kumar R 1995 The impact of postnatal depression on boys' intellectual development. Journal of Child Psychology and Psychiatry 36:1315–1337

Stewart-Brown S 1998 Emotional well-being and its relation to health. British Medical Journal 317:1608–1609

Stowe Z N, Nemeroff C B 1995 Women at risk for postpartum-onset major depression. American Journal of Obstetrics and Gynecology 173(2):639–645

Teti D M, Gelfand C M, Messinger D S, Isabella R 1995 Maternal depression and the quality of early attachment: an examination of infants, pre-schoolers and their mothers. Developmental Psychology 31:364–376

Udall E 1996 The childbirth conspiracy. Independent on Sunday (April 21) 73

Ullman S 1992 Fighting back: women's resistance to rape. Journal of Interpersonal Violence 7(1):62–80

Ward C 1995 Attitudes toward rape, feminist and social psychological perspectives. Sage, London

Whiffen V E 1988 Vulnerability to postpartum depression: a prospective multivariant study. Journal of Abnormal Psychology 97:467–474

Whitton A 1996 The pathway to care in postnatal depression: women's attitude to postnatal depression and its treatment. Midir's Midwifery Digest 7(1):93–94

Wickberg B, Hwang C P 1996 Counselling of postnatal depression: a controlled study on a population based Swedish sample. Journal of Affect Disorder 39:209–216

Young L 1998 Cute but dangerous. Guardian (November 11) 6

Zachary N, Stowe M D, Charles B, Nemeroff M 1995 Women at risk for postpartum-onset major depression. American Journal of Obstetrics and Gynecology 173(2):78–80

Recommended reading

Department of Health (DOH) 1998 Why mothers die – report on the confidential enquiries into maternal deaths in the United Kingdom 1994–1996. The Stationery Office, London

Reports on maternal deaths from suicide present a startling reality of the consequences of depression.

London Rape Crisis Centre (LRCC) 1992 Strength in numbers. LRCC, London

Madeson L 1994 Rebounding from childbirth, toward emotional recovery. Bergin & Garvey, Westport MA

Prescott-Clarke P, Primatesta P (eds) 1997 Health survey for England 1995: findings of a survey carried out on the behalf of the Department of Health, London. The Stationery Office, series HS(8), vol 1

Sharp D, Hay D, Pawlby S, Schmucher G, Allen H, Kumar R 1995 The impact of postnatal depression on boys' intellectual development. Journal of Child Psychology and Psychiatry 36:1315–1337

The consequences of postnatal depression, gender related. This paper explores the implications on the infant of a postnatally depressed mother.

Shipherd J, Beck J 1999 The effects of suppressing trauma-related thoughts on women with rape-related post-traumatic stress disorder. Behaviour Research and Therapy 37:99–112

Ward C 1995 Attitudes toward rape, feminist and social psychological perspectives. Sage, London

Challenges the reader's ideas about rape and sexual assault and explores the painful process of recovery.

Antenatal education leading the way for health promotion in midwifery

10

Overview

The aim of this chapter is to provide the reader with an opportunity to explore health education within the context of antenatal education. Teaching and learning will be explored from the perspective of empowering individuals to identify health needs and subsequently make informed choices. The long term consequences of antenatal education may enable participants to progress towards making healthy lifestyle choices. Raising awareness of health issues without increasing the potential for control or offering hope for future change may encourage feelings of frustration, negativity and powerlessness. Recognising the benefits of group support and the development of social networks is an integral part of the move toward personal autonomy and underpins the direction of the chapter. Although the focus of antenatal education throughout the following pages is related to education programmes and classes, the principles can be applied to one to one health education interactions during the antenatal, intrapartum and postnatal period. Principles discussed in Chapters 1 to 4 highlight problems associated with barriers to participation and strategies to enhance antenatal attendance.

Antenatal education – a strategy for health promotion

For health education to be effective it is important to consider the factors which influence how individuals behave, the socioeconomic context in which they conduct their everyday lives, what they want to learn and how they can achieve maximum learning. This will enable choices about childbirth experiences to be made. (Ch. 3 may provide further insight.) Today's maternity services are based on a philosophy which advocates informed choice and self-empowerment. Antenatal education is a window of opportunity for midwives to empower women and their families to be actively involved in developing decision-making skills in order to make choices. It is a fallacy to assume that the provision of information enables an individual to make an informed choice. This idea assumes that individuals have the necessary skills to be able to make informed decisions. The process of decision making is complex and is largely determined by individuals' thinking framework and their individual life experiences. Socioeconomic disadvantage influences to a large extent individual freedom to make choices about attendance to and participation in decisions about healthy lifestyle choices. Antenatal education which adopts a client-centred approach has the potential to begin the process of empowerment, which may influence other aspects of the individual's life beyond the postpartum period. Integral to this approach is the enhancement of communication and assertiveness skills, which may help to reduce professional boundaries, thus enabling further choice. Adopting a client-centred approach challenges the midwife's role as antenatal teacher and forces the adoption of the facilitative approach to learning. The interaction between the midwife and the client becomes limited to an area where the needs of the client and the expertise of the midwife overlap, thereby protecting the client from alien values. Traditionally antenatal education programmes have been prescribed by the midwife. This approach has been criticised for not meeting the individual needs of the client (Nolan 1998, Okpala 1991, Schott & Priest 1991). Hillan (1992) states that the teaching in antenatal classes did not prepare women adequately for labour or for parenthood. This is further supported by O'Meara (1993) and Nolan (1998) who suggest that parents are often disappointed with the poor preparation for parenthood and care of the newborn they receive. The ideas of Rogers & Freiberg (1994) are thought provoking and further challenge traditional antenatal education. They include the assertion that individuals should not be asked to learn something in which they see no personal relevance. Adults learn most effectively when they identify their own learning needs (Ewles & Simnett 1999).

The traditional approach to antenatal education can therefore be challenged. Effort should be directed toward identifying the needs and priorities of the woman and her partner, if present, and the formulation of objectives based on the needs identified. In an attempt to reach out to women who did not attend parenting classes Nicky Leap (1991) developed a weekly drop-in group based in a community centre which was open to women at any stage of their pregnancy. The group decided the contents of the sessions and the midwife facilitated group discussions, offered information if the need arose and helped new mothers who joined the group settle in. The women not only learned from each other but also developed personal growth by sharing information and supporting each other; they developed a form of social support, which continued beyond the postnatal period (Leap 1991).

The midwife as a facilitator of learning

I know I cannot teach anyone anything. I can only provide an environment in which he can learn.

Rogers & Freiberg (1994)

Providing an environment which is conducive to learning involves more than the physical changes one makes to the environment including the arrangement of chairs and removing perceived barriers to participation. It involves creating an environment which fosters a culture based on personal and group; growth, development, flexibility and trust. To provide this environment an appreciation of how adults learn is essential, and encourages the adoption of a teaching style which facilitates learning. A teacher who is directive, makes decisions about what should be learned and leaves little room for the value of human experience adopts the authoritarian approach to teaching. This style restricts participation and fosters an environment of power for the teacher. A demarcation between the professional's knowledge and the lay person's lack of knowledge is clearly defined. Clients may not feel able to disclose thoughts and feelings freely, possibly owing to the fear of being wrong, or from their perception that participation is not permitted. Adopting a participative style to learning is conducive to the role of a facilitator. A participative approach encourages growth and development of the client. The facilitator aids the learning process, and encourages a culture where self-discovery, self-action and self-determination are the focus for learning. What clients learn on their own through self-discovery is purported to be learned more deeply and permanently than what they are taught through formal methods (Ewles & Simnett 1999). Pertinent skills of a facilitator include: trust, flexibility, impartiality, empathy and an ability to deal with conflict appropriately. Rogers & Freiberg (1994) compare the role of the facilitator and the teacher and consider traditional teaching to be an overrated futile exercise (Box 10.1).

Box 10.1 **The roles of the teacher and the facilitator**

Teacher	Facilitator
Thinks of ways to teach effectively	Asks the group members what they want to learn
Decides content	Enquires about problems the group wishes to solve
Thinks of ways to help the participants learn more effectively	Thinks of resources the group may use to enhance learning
	Uses strategies which enable participants to learn from experience, and each other

Box 10.2 **The first antenatal class**

Firn welcomed the prospective parents at the entrance to the antenatal education room. She had prepared the room so that the environment was informal and inviting, despite worn carpet and low uncomfortable chairs. Chairs were arranged in a circle. As each participant arrived they were invited to write their names on a sticky label. After a general welcome by herself, Firn divided the class into groups of four and asked them to talk amongst themselves for 5 minutes, finding out three things about each other including names. She did not prescribe the other two items. Firn joined a group and took part in the activity. She then asked each group of four to join the neighbouring group of four and asked them to share the information they had gained, introducing each other. This activity was repeated once more until the introductions extended to the whole group. Firn then offered a coffee break and asked the participants to think about what they would like to discuss over the following weeks. After coffee, she gave each original group of four a flip chart and pen and asked them to write down what they felt they would like to discuss during the following weeks. Firn displayed the flip charts on the walls and encouraged the group to participate in placing the contents into an acceptable order for the following weeks. The group chose one subject that they wanted to discuss that week.

Reflection points

- Which teaching style has Firn utilised?
- What improvements could Firn have made?

Some educators may use the strengths of the two approaches to maximise the learning opportunity. Empowerment is a fundamental aspect of the participative approach to learning and cannot be adopted using authoritarian styles. Although becoming a facilitator involves risk taking and an ability to deal with uncertainties and difficulties, it enables deep and meaningful learning to take place (Rogers & Freiberg 1994).

As an example of the difference between the two styles, consider Box 10.2.

Learning – an insight

Miller (1994) refers to learning as a purposeful activity which often results in a change in a person's thinking, behaviour or both. It can be argued that learning is not always purposeful and may be incidental. Incidental learning is more likely to occur if the learning process is facilitated rather than controlled. The aim of understanding how adults learn involves the utilisation of teaching methods which will enhance the learning process. It is every midwife's intent, be it during one to one teaching or during group teaching, that clients will:

- learn something new
- enhance their existing knowledge
- raise their awareness
- learn a skill
- reflect on previous experiences
- encourage the exploration of attitudes and beliefs
- reinforce or dispel myths
- challenge stereotypes
- feel able to make decisions.

Antenatal groups generally consist of many different people from varying social and cultural groups. Each person has individual ways of learning or processing information. The majority will learn by thinking, feeling and doing. The taxonomy of educational objectives as proposed by Bloom (1956) are referred to by Miller (1994), as 'learning domains' and are categorised into the cognitive domain (thinking), the affective domain (feeling) and the psychomotor domain (doing). When planning antenatal education and setting aims and objectives it is useful to decide the domain in which the client will focus most time and energy in order to achieve the maximum learning potential. If the aim of the session is to explore attitudes toward breast feeding then the affective domain is the area where most learning is likely to take place. The method chosen for learning would therefore reflect this. Prior thought should also be given to cognitive and psychomotor domains, if learning about breast feeding is to be meaningful.

The cognitive domain

Cognition is concerned with thinking. It is a process which involves exploring a thought in the mind, making sense of things, accepting, refuting, recalling and making inferences. Learners may simply know the facts but be unable to make sense of them, or they may be able to understand them but be unable to apply them. Critical thinking, problem solving and creative thinking can be facilitated to encourage the application of new knowledge.

The affective domain

Affective in this context refers to feelings or emotions; it reflects attitudes and belief systems. It is by far the most difficult of the three domains to measure owing to its individual, subjective nature. However, it is extremely beneficial when teaching emotive subjects, or any subject which creates a mental block for a participant who is emotionally distressed about a particular experience. To deliver the programme without considering this domain may achieve superficial, limited learning, or possibly no learning at all.

Consider the scenario in Box 10.3. Daphne did not hear what the midwife was saying about breast feeding. She had set her agenda before she arrived at the session and felt confident at the end of the session that she would have the right approach to feeding her baby this time. Adopting a different approach to teaching, including participation, exploration of thoughts and feelings, may have influenced a different outcome.

The psychomotor domain

This is concerned with doing, or performing a skill, procedure or behaviour. This type of learning lends itself to many subjects taught during the

---

Box 10.3 Case scenario: Daphne

Daphne arrived at the parenting session on breast feeding with preconceived ideas about how she would feed her baby. She had already made up her mind that she was going to breast and bottle feed her newborn as she had done this with her previous child Tommy, who is now a thriving 4 year old. The antenatal education session consisted of a short lecture on breast feeding followed by a video which repeated the content of the lecture. Group participation was not encouraged and the group were not asked to contribute their thoughts, feelings or ideas. During the lecture, as the midwife informed the group of the advantages and disadvantages of breast feeding, Daphne reflected back on her previous experience:

'I know I'll be topping up this baby with formulae feed; if I'd have done that sooner with Tommy he wouldn't have ended up losing weight and crying all the time. He must have been starving, the poor thing. You must give the bottle feed as well as the breast because the breast cannot fill up big babies.'

At the end of the lecture Daphne summarised her own thoughts:

'I'll do it right this time around, the right thing for all of us.'

antenatal period and is by far the easiest to measure. Facilitating learning of positions in labour to prospective parents is an obvious example. The midwife would show the clients how to adopt and maintain certain positions, or indeed ask clients if they are familiar with any positions in labour that they could share with the group. The facilitator could take part and share experiences of different positions which may support and help the birth process using relevant research-based evidence. Repetition can only seek to enhance learning and is an active part of this domain. This may move toward the activity being performed without guidance from the facilitator. The client may progress toward adapting the positions learned to suit different circumstances to those taught, including, for example, comfortable positions for the antenatal period or positions that ease backache.

As you have probably concluded at this stage, effective utilisation of the three domains can be achieved only through recognition of the interdependent relationship among the domains. Teaching a group of clients a skill should not occur without encouraging cognition and the exploration of thoughts and feelings. Similarly Rogers & Freiberg (1994) refer to whole person learning which involves thinking, feeling and doing but also includes intuition and experience. Whole person learning aids memory retention owing to its depth and scope. Adults who learn new information antenatally or clarify misconceptions hope to remember their new-found knowledge. Short term memory has a limited capacity, however, Miller (1994) suggests that only five to seven thoughts can be held in short term memory at any one time. Antenatal education should therefore be offered in short intervals to avoid overbombarding participants with information. Slavin (1988) suggests that participants will retain less if the latter occurs. It is suggested that information received is scanned for significance and personal meaning and then ranked according to how it will be remembered. If it is considered important it will be retained in the long term memory. Long term memory has no known limit to its capacity. Information will be stored in the long term memory if the person is receptive and if it is of personal use to the recipient. Memory retention is also influenced by other factors including the quality of the information received, the methods used for its delivery and the circumstances under which the information is received (Child 1993).

Teaching methods

A worthwhile education programme should be well supported with appropriate teaching methods. During the planning stages of antenatal education, consideration of the following points may enable the utilisation of appropriate teaching methods:

- methods that will assist the achievement of the learning objectives
- methods that will maximise learning
- methods that enhance memory retention
- methods that maintain interest
- thought-provoking methods.

Lecture method

The lecture method is predominantly teacher led. The teacher usually imparts information to a group of people. Interaction is usually limited to questions posed by the teacher to the group, or a member of the group asking questions. The group's main activity therefore, is listening or taking notes. One main advantage of the lecture method is the ability to communicate information to a large number of people. The midwife may use this method to direct factual information to a group of clients. This method may then be supported by group work/discussion, which serves to encourage a deeper more meaningful understanding of the content. The lecture method has reduced in popularity in antenatal education as it is less effective than other methods for encouraging the sharing of ideas and exploration of thoughts and feelings.

Making the lecture enjoyable

If the lecture method is chosen, it is important to remember that the average person's attention span is 20 minutes, after which time there is a reduction in the amount of information assimilated (Quinn 1995). During pregnancy, however, this time is reduced to 10 minutes (Schott & Priest 1991). The lecture therefore should be short, sharp and directly to the point, presenting information in a logical clear format to promote maximum assimilation. The format presented in Table 10.1 (p. 213) may be a useful guide to enable a logical presentation of information. Repetition should be used frequently so that the group hears the information more than once. This approach enables the group to retain the information for longer. Antenatal education presents many challenges for the midwife, who may be requested to cover wide and varied subjects during a limited period of time. The programme should be primarily decided by the client group and a structure for delivery agreed between the group and the midwife. The lecture method may be utilised to save time since other methods which are predominantly student led take longer. Participation should be encouraged, however, as this helps to maintain the group's level of arousal and interest. Encouraging group members to share their experiences provides a valuable and interesting learning opportunity for other members of the group. Life experiences, which are usually expressed with a degree of emotion, are likely to be remembered by group members. Asking questions and encouraging the group to ask questions is an example of group participation.

Questions may encourage the group to think critically about a particular approach to care, assess the knowledge base, encourage the group's orientation to learning and demonstrate interest and value. The midwife should ensure that participants feel able to ask questions during the lecture. (See section on Group dynamics, p. 217.) Some midwives, however, may prefer questions to be saved until the end of the lecture. To maximise the response to questioning, the midwife should aim to keep her questions simple and preferably open ended. For example:

- Can anyone in the group share their experiences of…?
- Can you describe how that made you feel when…?
- Can anyone share any positive things about…?
- What are your positive thoughts about childbirth…?

(Note that closed questions invite one-word answers.)

Group work

Problem-solving groups

This type of group work encourages critical thinking and aids memory retention through problem association. To be meaningful, the problem to be solved should be appropriate and relevant to the potential experiences of the participants. As memory works through association (Knowles, Holton & Swanson 1998), this approach enables the development and retention of the problem-solving process. Participants are able to take chances based on the decisions they make about a particular problem or scenario, within a secure and safe environment. Decision-making skills may also be developed during this activity. Working through a problem in this situation requires knowledge, critical thought and discussion. Once the problem has been solved participants may feel a degree of confidence and satisfaction. This may aid memory retention and ownership of the problem solved. The process of solving the problem would undoubtedly aid learning. The problem may require one answer or a range of answers and this will be determined by the objectives. This technique requires careful preparation and planning. The aim of the activity and the problem should be clearly defined prior to the start of the activity.

Buzz groups

Buzz groups are useful interesting ways of encouraging two or more people to come together to discuss a particular aspect of the session. Alternatively, the participants may be asked to write down everything they know about a subject based on their existing knowledge, thoughts and life experiences. This information may then be shared with other members of the group – either verbally or by a self-nominated member of the group reading the ideas from the flip chart. (The facilitator may choose to take on this role if group members are not willing.) Participants who do not wish to write on a flip chart should be given the option of presenting their information verbally. An appropriate time limit should be allocated.

The facilitator may also encourage one buzz group (group one) to join with another (group two) to share ideas and opinions and then feed back to the main group. Or, group one and two may be asked to join with another buzz group (group three); this is commonly known as 'snowballing'. Eventually all the original buzz groups (for example, groups one, two and three), conclude as one big group, each having shared their ideas and opinions with each other (see Box 10.2). This is a very good process for encouraging all group members to participate in the activity and also encourages the participants to interact with each other. Group members who may feel intimidated and lack confidence when speaking out in a large group may feel more comfortable when contributing to a small buzz group.

Brainstorming

'Brainstorming' is exactly what the name suggests. The idea is for each member of the group to generate as many ideas as possible about a given problem situation, method or procedure. One of the ground rules here is that there should be no criticism regardless of the nature of the response. The facilitator, or a volunteer from the group, may write down the responses on a flip chart. Note, however, that responses will be forthcoming only if the original instruction is clear and focused and the environment enables free expression of thoughts and ideas. A safe environment will ultimately influence the nature of the response (see Group dynamics). Once the brainstorming session is complete it must be summarised, evaluated, commended and utilised within the next part of the session, or used to complete the session.

Discussion

If the discussion method is facilitated appropriately it will encourage the sharing of ideas, thoughts, opinions and experiences of a subject and very often involves emotions, which may include elation, excitement, sadness and anger. The discussion method is concerned with student-centred learning. The focus is on the group participants. The facilitator becomes a passive observer but facilitates the discussion, by acknowledging, agreeing, encouraging, sharing, accepting and/or refuting. Although this method is an enriching and fruitful approach to learning, it is by far one of the most difficult to initiate and maintain if the group does not feel able to disclose or offer opinions and thoughts freely. The discussion method should be utilised once the group members are working well together. Facilitation of this process is highlighted in the section on promoting positive group dynamics.

The facilitator may decide how long the discussion will run, with some degree of flexibility. If the discussion raises pertinent points and the participants, through expression of both verbal and non-verbal behaviour, appear to be enjoying the process, then the facilitator may decide to let the discussion last for longer than previously planned. Some authors suggest that the discussion should take as long as it needs (Nolan 1998, Rogers & Freiberg 1994). The facilitator, together with the group participants, should have decided the content of the discussion prior to its start.

There are a number of pitfalls, however. First, it is possible that if the discussion continues for the duration of the class then some group participants may feel cheated because the subject they wished to discuss, or receive some information about, would not be covered. Others enter the antenatal class expecting the sessions to be teacher led. Because of their preconceived ideas about education, they arrive at the class expecting to be taught (Knowles 1990). The benefits of a discussion which may appear to monopolise the session may, therefore, not be recognised. This may be more apparent during free-discussion groups where the subject for discussion is chosen by the group and under the control of group members. Prior to the commencement of the antenatal class, therefore, it is important that the midwife explains the educational approach that will be taken and its significance.

Adopting varied teaching methods, with the support of learning aids, can help to maximise each group participant's learning experience.

Starting a discussion – a useful example

Consider the scenario in Box 10.4.

Clear aims and objectives for a discussion should be established prior to its start. Consideration should be given to the trigger for the discussion. In the scenario in Box 10.4 a video was used as a trigger for stimulating a discussion. Videos can be useful aids for this purpose (see Visual aids below), but it may be useful if the facilitator has a list of preset open-ended questions concerning the video which can be offered to the group to enhance the discussion. This approach may, however, focus the discussion toward the facilitator's personal agenda. Raising issues about the video, or offering consideration pointers, may also be useful. Ultimately the aims and objectives should determine the nature of the discussion.

A single command like, 'Now let's have a discussion' is open to interpretation, and poses questions to the group participants which may include:

'A discussion about what aspect, what point?'
'Does the midwife want us to offer our opinions about pain relief in general, or discuss what we thought about the video?'

Ambiguous requests cause confusion and may encourage a silent response.

Box 10.4 **Antenatal education class**

Immediately after showing a video which described the different methods of pain relief and involved women talking about their experiences, Faith said to the group:

'Now lets have a discussion.'

This was followed by 30 seconds of silence. Faith began to get a little nervous and posed another question:

'Has anybody got any thoughts they would like to share?'

This was again followed by 30 seconds of silence. Then one woman shared her previous experience of using TENS for pain relief and the group listen attentively. This then triggered another woman to tell the group about her sister's experience of using the epidural as a form of pain relief. Both women had briefly shared accounts of two pain relief methods. No reference was made toward the content of the video.

Faith felt relieved that two people had shared their experiences, but felt uncomfortable about facilitating future discussions. She thanked them for sharing their experiences and moved on to the second part of the session, the subject of which was non-pharmacological methods of pain relief.

Reflection points

- Did a discussion take place?
- Was the aim of using the visual aid achieved?
- Consider ways in which the situation could have been improved

Alternatively, in a well-planned discussion where group members participate freely, well-meaning individuals who feel the need to share all their experiences may present their whole life stories, thus dominating the discussion and inhibiting others from taking part. Reminding the group of the preset ground rules may prevent this situation from happening again, or reduce its occurrence. The facilitator may interject at an appropriate time by thanking the individual for her contribution and include other group members by asking them to share a different or similar experience. A timely interjection may also be an appropriate moment to encourage others to participate by emphasising the benefits of sharing different experiences and opinions. The more opinions and experiences that are offered the more fruitful the discussion will be. The aims and objectives of each parenting session will, to a large extent, determine the teaching methods. The content of Table 10.1 will help you to choose an appropriate teaching method against the objectives set. (You may in fact have more than one aim but for the purpose of this exercise only one aim is stated.)

Visual aids

Appropriate use of visual aids or teaching materials serves many purposes, some of which include giving meaning to abstract concepts, bringing understanding to complicated subjects by appealing to sensory powers of

Table 10.1
Teaching methods for particular aims and objectives

Subject requested	Aim	Objectives	Teaching method
Signs of onset of labour	To explore different signs and symptoms which may indicate that labour is starting	Discuss personal ideas about the onset of labour Identify signs of the onset of labour	Buzz groups, brainstorm
		Develop decision-making skills including when to call the midwife Empowered to make decisions	Lecture, small group activity, e.g. case studies, picture form or written record Small group activity e.g. problem solving
When things go wrong in labour, complications	Raise awareness of the reasons why complications occur during labour and the mode of action taken to alleviate problems	Discuss personal ideas about what could go wrong Understand the main principles behind interventions used to alleviate complications Be involved in the decision-making process if things do not go according to plan during labour	Buzz groups, brainstorm Lecture, discussion and exploration of pre-set appropriate scenarios Small group work, problem-solving activities
Sexual intercourse before and after birth	To explore ideas about sex during pregnancy and the postnatal period	Confirm and/or dispel ideas about sex during pregnancy Explore attitudes and belief systems Feel empowered to make choices	Buzz groups, discussion Group work, discussion
Pelvic floor exercises	To raise awareness of the importance of performing pelvic floor exercise	Understand the importance of this activity Carry out pelvic floor exercises Discuss strategies which will assist in compliance	Lecture Demonstration with model (see Ch. 8) Buzz groups

Table 10.1 (cont'd)	Subject requested	Aim	Objectives	Teaching method
	Positions in labour	To raise awareness about the benefits of adopting different positions in labour	Examine personal feelings about alternative positions	Discussion groups
			Discuss the advantages and disadvantages of alternative positions	Small lecture
			Adopt different positions which could be used antenatally and during the labour period	Discussion of written or picture scenarios, demonstration

seeing and/or feeling. The range of visual aids is endless, but financial resources very often limit the number available. Those commonly used include videos, models, posters, flip charts and photographs. Handouts and leaflets are also popular and enable the client to access and utilise the information at their own pace. Using visual aids which require literacy ability may, however, create barriers to participation and impede the learning process for those who are illiterate or for those whose first language is not represented. Using a combination of visual aids which do not all require literacy skills may help to reduce the barrier to participation and learning.

The video is considered to be the closest substitute to the actual experience (Miller 1994). When used as a visual aid, overreliance should be avoided. Depending on its length and content, it is not essential that the video is shown in its entirety. Certain parts can be viewed to generate responses and create a discussion. The video may also be stopped temporarily at a certain point to provide the opportunity for discussion, to answer certain questions, to highlight particular points relevant to the objectives of the session or to enable the group to discuss favourable endings based on their knowledge, thoughts and opinions.

The pelvis – a commonly used visual aid

Midwives have for many years developed their own visual aids or utilised one model to illustrate many different subject areas. The pelvic model is often used for this purpose. Box 10.5 shows how it may be used as a visual aid for a range of subjects.

The development of a poster, model or activity could also be effective

Box 10.5 **The pelvic model used as a visual aid**

Labour

1. Teaching basic anatomy – What is the pelvis? Where is it? (launching straight into a session on labour without discussing the pelvis is like building a house without foundations)
2. Functions of the pelvis – What does it do?
3. Changes which occur as a result of pregnancy and labour
4. The mechanism of labour

Teaching pelvic floor exercises (see Ch. 8)

Visual association of the area concerned with pelvic floor exercises can supplement verbal description and enhance correct compliance. The pelvic model may therefore:

5. Establish the location of the pelvic floor muscles
6. Illustrate the pelvic floor muscles and their function

Adopting different positions in labour

Visual representation of the pelvic model when, for example, the body is in the all-fours position demonstrates the change in position of the pelvis, which aids understanding. The pelvic model may therefore be used to:

7. Demonstrate the change in the position of the pelvis, prior to individual participation and practice of different positions which may be adopted in labour

When things go wrong

If there is a request to discuss this subject, the pelvic model may be used to illustrate (with the aid of a doll), for example:

8. Prolonged labour and possible reasons, e.g. malposition

and does not require professional finishing. Despite the benefits of using visual aids, care should be taken, however, that they are not used as a substitute for the facilitator.

The use of audiotapes – a useful example

Audiocassette tapes are useful for the development of skills including relaxation and exercise. They may also be used to assist the midwife to teach breathing awareness. It is not an unusual request for a midwife to be asked to teach how breathing can be used as a coping mechanism during labour. Some midwives may choose to simulate the expression of pain (whimpering, heavy sighing and breathing, facial expressions of pain, etc.) experienced during a contraction whilst demonstrating several different patterns of breathing which may be used as a coping strategy. However, others may feel uncomfortable about simulating this activity within an antenatal class. In this case, audiotapes can be extremely useful. The simulation could be audiotaped outside of the education forum by a willing colleague, for example, which would provide the midwife with an audiotaped version of expressions of pain. The audio tape may in addition have a narrator, indicating when the contraction starts, when it becomes more painful and when it ends, added into the sequence of expression of pain in each stage – through heavy sighs, whimpers and cries which increase in intensity as the contraction becomes stronger. During the antenatal education session the midwife would simply demonstrate breathing techniques at the start of, during and toward the end of the taped verbal expression of contraction pain. The tape could be repeated and participation invited.

Taking your colleague's class – tips for success

The ideal situation is that midwives are at all times prepared to facilitate antenatal education; this, however, is not always the case. On rare occasions midwives are asked to facilitate an antenatal class at short notice. It is also not uncommon for a midwife to be required to inform a client on a one to one basis about a particular aspect of care or drug so that an informed decision can be made. Whatever the circumstance, the prime objective is to ensure understanding. The provision of clear, focused and accurate information is a good starting point. Midwives should ask themselves the following questions if the content of the session or interaction is to be delivered effectively.

- What is the aim (what do you want to do)?
- What are the objectives (what do you hope the clients will achieve)?
- What method will you use to achieve this?
- How will you gauge the depth of the content?
- How will you assess levels of understanding and learning?

You may choose to categorise the subject into seven small sections. For instance, consider the following questions and use pethidine as an example of the subject you are asked to teach.

1. What is it, or what is it like?
2. What does it do or what happens?
3. What are the advantages?
4. What are the disadvantages?
5. How do you do it, use it, promote it, prevent it, etc.?
6. Does the subject warrant talking about side-effects? If so, include them.
7. What are the alternatives?

These questions will lend themselves to most subjects, for example: pain relief in labour, positions in labour, first stage of labour, second stage of labour, methods of third stage delivery, breast feeding, bottle feeding, relaxation, exercise, vitamin K, sudden infant death syndrome, etc. This list is not intended to be prescriptive but is intended to help those midwives who have been given very short notice to facilitate an antenatal class.

Group dynamics

When facilitating antenatal education how often have you thought that something was not quite right with the way the group worked together? How often have you said, 'I can't put my finger on it, but something is just not right'? The reasons why questions of this nature arise are wide and varied. The aim here is not to work through the intricate webs of intuitive thought. Exploring the issues apparent when groups of different people are brought together and expected to perform certain tasks, learn a particular task, discuss issues, build social networks, become empowered to make decisions or make lifestyle changes is far more beneficial. Whatever the expectation of the class, both from the facilitator's and the participants' perspective, the dynamics of the group that they become a part of influences the knowledge, depth and experience that each participant takes away. The aim of understanding group dynamics is to enable groups to work to their full potential, thereby achieving not only the aims of the group but also the personal and individual aims of all participants. Positive group dynamics is determined to a large extent on how the group is facilitated. All group members share common characteristics with their neighbours; they also share similar aims and objectives. People generally attend antenatal education because they wish to:

- learn something new
- receive reassuring information
- reinforce what they know already by seeking out others to evaluate the accuracy of personal beliefs and attitudes (Festinger 1950)
- clarify issues of concern
- meet other people to satisfy interpersonal needs.

What is group dynamics?

Kurt Lewin (1951) coined this phrase and is widely recognised as the 'parent' of group dynamics. Lewin (1953) refers to groups as being powerful, active, fluid and catalysing, as opposed to being weak, passive and static. Forsyth (1990 p. 13), summarised group dynamics as being both the 'powerful processes that influence individuals when in group situations and the study of these processes'.

Group Development

Many theorists over the last century have assumed that groups pass through several stages as they develop. Understanding the stages of development may enhance the facilitator's ability to support the process of development without feeling a sense of failure during tension and conflict moments. Tuckman labelled the stages forming, storming, norming, performing and adjourning (Tuckman 1965, Tuckman & Jenson 1977). Forsyth (1990) describes the stages in more detail and suggests that when groups meet they first need to orientate themselves to each other (forming); secondly, they may find themselves in conflict as they meet individual differences of attitudes and beliefs, ideas and opinions (storming); thirdly, norms and roles may start to develop which seek to modify behaviour and encourage group unity (norming); fourthly, the group may reach a stage where it can perform as a unit and is fully functional to achieve the aims of the group (performing). The last stage is concerned with the group reaching a state where it can dissolve as the aim of the group is achieved and the task is completed (adjourning).

Forming

When groups meet they need to orientate themselves to each other. Consider the scenario in Box 10.6. In this, the five individual groups of three have a task to complete. Not all group members know each other. Some may feel as though they have been placed together with a group of strangers. Some may feel that they would like to contribute their thoughts but feel that their requests may be viewed as being too simplistic by other group members. Others may feel that, by revealing their real requests, they will

Box 10.6 **Scenario 1, part 1**

A collection of people are sitting in the antenatal education room waiting for the first class to start. From the records it is established that they are all very different not only by occupation but also by ethnic origin, social class and the very obvious age and gender differences. The group consists of couples, women who arrive alone, others who have arrived with a friend in tow and a few men who arrive alone. There are a total of 15 people in the room. After a general introduction by the midwife (see section on 'ice melters'), the group is divided into groups of three. The participants are asked to discuss what they would like to cover during the following weeks and why. The midwife requests that this information is recorded on a flip chart by a volunteer from each group and presented to the large group. The groups are not forthcoming with their requests; some contribute, some sit in silence whilst others talk to their partners. Those who have attended alone try to direct their gaze away from everybody.

Reflection point

- What could the midwife have done to prevent this situation from happening?

Box 10.7 **Scenario 1, part 2**

The midwife observes the small group interaction and attempts to rescue the situation. Coffee is brought in as the groups work and the midwife decides to rotate the flip charts around so that each group has another group's flip chart, to continue with their list of requests for the programme. The small groups have coffee whilst spending another 10 minutes together.

As the flip charts are rotated, the small group members observe the contributions of the other groups. Identification and familiarity of what is written on the flip chart is reassuring for some members of the group, whilst others feel reassured that participants from the other groups had requested the same things. Some tension is therefore dispelled and the initial inhibitions that arose from interaction with strangers subsides. Exchange of information flows more freely about members' aims and expectations of the course and themselves.

The midwife then rotates the flip charts again and asks for any additional contributions to be made. The original groups stay together for a further 5 minutes. They begin to function as groups and not individuals. Finally, a volunteer from each small group relays the information contained on the final flip chart to the whole group.

reveal their personal views and values and expose personal feelings of vulnerability. Leery (1983) suggests that some people believe that they lack the social skills necessary to cope with the situation and actively choose to avoid group membership.

The scenario continues in Box 10.7, as the midwife introduces some strategies to remedy the lack of interaction.

Storming

As the course progresses, the group moves toward being at the limit of the politeness and orientation stage. Some group members may now feel able to resist, disagree, disrupt, destruct or challenge. Conflict is accepted as a developmental process and therefore a positive aspect of group formation. It is suggested (Bales, Cohen & Williamson 1979) that conflict is as common as group harmony and disagreement is a natural consequence of joining a group. Low levels of conflict in a group indicate that group members are uninvolved, bored and unmotivated (Forsyth 1990). A certain amount of conflict can help a group to function well and to a certain extent determines the stability of the group. It can resolve tension, clarify unspoken misunderstandings and re-establish unity. Conversely, conflict that is not expressed can invariably cause tension within a group to the extent that non-verbal behaviour and unaired hostilities divide a group and render the group dysfunctional, and not capable of reaching its acquired goal.

Box 10.8 **Example of a conflict situation in antenatal education**

An overzealous member of the group who is extremely knowledgeable constantly has an overwhelming urge to express information which is not only up to date but, as she informs the other group members, 'hot off the press, retrieved from the Internet'. Small group discussions are dominated and controlled by this person who feels that her contribution is not only valid but essential for the group. If others dare to offer an opinion they may be interrupted, 'corrected' and challenged by this group member. Another group member who is equally passionate about childbirth expresses an expert knowledge in the area, and constantly seeks to challenge the first. These two overzealous group members dominate group discussion and render any learning which may have taken place obsolete.

The facilitator can be instrumental in preventing escalating conflict – that is, where one area of conflict leads into another. An example is described in Box 10.8.

The storming described in Box 10.8 could be extremely disruptive for the group as it involves only two members. Other group members may collude to support one or either member, or they may choose to withdraw themselves from the group. The facilitator can reduce the conflict by incorporating the following strategies to inhibit this monopolisation of the session.

• Refer the group back to the ground rules, for example: 'do not interrupt whilst others are speaking', 'value each others' contributions'.
• Place both individuals in the same group so they are working together to achieve the same goal.
• Inform them that, although their contributions are greatly valued, it is important that other group members are given the opportunity to contribute equally in order for the group to function to its full potential.
• Encourage them to print out their findings and share them with the group at the end of the session or during coffee break instead of verbalising them throughout the session.

Conflict can also be reduced through negotiation skills which are based on the principled negotiator, as proposed by Fisher & Wry (1981).

The midwife could:

• emphasise that the goal was set by the group to be reached efficiently and amicably
• separate the people from the problem
• focus on the interests of the group and not on the different positions
• create options for mutual gain
• attempt to reach a result based on standards and not on individual will.

Norming

Group members at this stage should be able to sense a feeling of unity, stability, ownership and membership. Interdependence is very much a feature of this stage of group development. There are lower levels of anxiety and increasing pressure for conformity. The group on the whole becomes more cohesive and has greater control over those group members who challenged the established group norm. The two individuals who increased conflict in the group in Box 10.8 would, at this stage, be performing within the group, for the group and not performing as individuals. They would be reallocated roles by the group where they could continue with their passion for knowledge. This would continue not at the expense of destroying the group but through strategies that were enabling and supportive.

It has been highlighted, however, that groups which are too cohesive can be destructive. If the norm for the group is underperformance then the control exerted over all group members will be a negative disabling approach. Cohesion can also lead to scapegoating and rejection (Wolf 1985).

Performing

At this stage the group will be able to work toward achieving the goal. It will function to its full potential. The group members will be able to deal with emotive and sensitive subjects – like, for example, sudden infant death syndrome, complications during labour and sex during pregnancy – and feel as though they had achieved their overall aim. In contrast, some groups may remain in the conflict stage, which prevents the group from working to its full potential. Groups that have passed through the stages of forming, storming, norming and performing are more productive at dealing with issues that require a high coordination of effort. In contrast, groups who remain in the storming stage may attend the session and contribute from an individual's point of view toward achieving the overall goal but find group work which requires a high coordination of effort difficult. There is no guarantee that the group which has progressed through the stages as described by Tuckman (Tuckman 1965, Tuckman & Jenson 1977) will perform effectively, especially if, as mentioned above, the group norm is underperformance. At the performance stage, nevertheless, groups are more enjoyable and foster a sense of safety and group identity, which are vital ingredients towards a productive learning culture. Once the group members are performing well together, the facilitator may request that they divide into smaller groups, where they have the opportunity to work with others with whom they have had little contact. This will encourage group identity and reduce the powerful influences of subgroups.

Although group behaviour may involve norming and storming before actually performing, not all groups may reach the performance stage by progressing in a linear fashion as Tuckman describes. Groups may return to the conflict stage or even to the norming stage when faced with particular issues before maximum performance can be reached. Some groups avoid certain stages and still manage to achieve the desired goal. Some theorists (Hill & Gruner 1973, Shambaugh 1978) prefer the cyclical models of group development whereby a group may cycle through the developmental stages as determined by Tuckman (1965), and return to the same issues (e.g. conflict) later in the group's life. Returning to one of the developmental stages would enable the group members to revisit that stage with previous knowledge of their original experience. The group would therefore have a heightened sense of internal protection of its individual members and thus not exhibit the same degree of conflict that occurred prior to group members knowing each other.

Adjourning

This stage can be quite difficult to deal with. Very often antenatal education that is taking place in the hospital environment has a planned adjournment stage. The programme completes and the next group starts. Despite the well-known benefits of antenatal groups continuing (Leap 1991), most hospital resources at present do not accommodate ongoing antenatal groups. Community groups may disband the adjournment stage and continue the group with a new agenda. The adjournment stage can be stressful for members who feel a loss of group support. The facilitator may encourage group members to maintain contact. Others will need no encouragement and establish group networks.

Reflection points

- Reflect on the group dynamics of a group you have observed, or are currently a member of.
- Did the group progress through the stages of group development as described by Tuckman?
- How did the group develop towards the performance stage?
- What was the role of the facilitator throughout the stages of group development?

Involving partners

Discussing the nature of the partner's or birth attendant's role enables clarity of role responsibility and fosters a sense of belonging and participation in the birth process. Exploring hopes and fears can very often clarify roles that will be undertaken and acknowledges those which may pose problems. A survey carried out by Szeverenyi, Poka & Rorok (1998) explored childbirth-related fears among a sample of 216 prospective parents. Over 80% of men expressed some fears relating to childbirth. They were particularly fearful of their wives having severe pain, an operative delivery, fetal birth injuries, helplessness, powerlessness or dying during childbirth; 76% felt that their presence at delivery would have no adverse effect on their future relationship with their wives. Identifying specific fears can enable discussion and enhance role clarity, thereby reducing the potential for spouse conflict. A study which sought to describe the experiences of fathers who were present during childbirth demonstrated the need for support and guidance for fathers during the intrapartum and postnatal period (Julkunen & Liukkonen 1998). Preparation through antenatal education may enable partners to progress through the birth and postnatal experience feeling empowered to be able to offer support. Raphael-Leff (1993) suggests that support offered by birth partners is more likely to be psychological and tactile in nature as opposed to birth coach. It is important to clarify role identity and responsibility during antenatal education. This will avoid disappointment and conflict. Midwives can facilitate group discussion, encouraging the disclosure of the partners' perceptions of their role. Prescribed roles should be avoided and myths and stereotypes about fatherhood challenged where appropriate. For births taking place in the hospital outside of the familiar home environment, the partner may feel that permission should be gained prior to carrying out supportive roles. Exploring this possibility during the antenatal period may work toward reducing such boundaries.

Points for consideration and discussion may include the following.

- The individual wants and needs of the partner
- The antenatal period – hopes and fears:
  - offering support – what is needed, what can be offered
  - change in partner's body image
  - sexual relationship
- Labour and delivery:
  - being present at the birth – hopes and fears
  - being absent during the birth
  - offering support – what is needed, what can be offered
    role identification
  - debriefing after the experience – exploration of thoughts and feelings
- Postnatal period and beyond:
  - parenthood – hopes and fears
  - developing parental roles
  - supporting each other – what is needed, what can be offered.

If the subject is not requested by group participants the midwife may choose to offer the points for consideration in the form of a handout to those who express an interest. If group work is undertaken to elicit hopes and fears it is important to remember that not all partners are male and, as such, an attempt should be made to avoid comments like, for example: 'Can we have all the fathers in this group?'

Evaluation

A valuable part of antenatal education is the evaluation. It may be performed during the class, at the end of the class or a considerable time after the programme has ended. The aim and nature of the evaluation will determine when and how it is carried out. It is useful for midwives to formalise methods of evaluation to enable audit and provision of data, which demonstrate the viability of the programme. Evaluating antenatal classes can reassure the facilitator that things are going well, or enable amendments to be made prior to the start of the subsequent class. Several aspects of the session can be evaluated and include evaluation of the facilitator, evaluation of learning and self-evaluation by the facilitator. (Evaluation is covered in detail in Ch. 11, and provides a complementary text to this brief overview.)

Evaluation of the teacher

You may find it useful to establish the following.

- Did they find you approachable?
- Did they find you audible?
- Did they find the session easy to follow?
- Did they enjoy the session?
- Do they think that there was anything that you could have done differently?

Evaluation of learning

You may find it useful to establish the following.

- What did they learn?
- Did they achieve the objectives set? How do you know this?
- Did they learn anything new?
- Do they feel that other subjects should have been covered?

Self-evaluation

You may find it useful to establish the following.

- What did I do well?
- Where could I have improved?
- Did I answer questions appropriately?
- Did the group work achieve the desired aim?
- Did I facilitate the discussion?
- Did I encourage all group members to take an active part in the session based on their individual abilities?
- Did I enjoy the session?
- Do I need to produce more comprehensive handouts?
- Did the handouts complement the session?
- Did I achieve the objectives set?
- Did I feel threatened at any time during the session?

Summary

- Antenatal education provides a window of opportunity for midwives to be proactive in influencing the adoption of healthy lifestyle choices, and through facilitation skills can enable women and their partners to make decisions about their care preferences.
- Education which is client centred encourages participation, values life experiences and invokes a sense of value for each group member.
- A worthwhile education programme should be well supported with appropriate teaching methods.
- Learning is a purposeful activity which often results in a change in a person's thinking, behaviour or both.
- The taxonomy of educational objectives is referred to as learning domains and is categorised into the cognitive domain (thinking), the affective domain (feeling) and the psychomotor domain (doing). When planning antenatal education and setting aims and objectives it is useful to decide in which domain the client will focus most time and energy, in order to achieve the maximum learning potential.
- Attention to group dynamics is worthwhile if antenatal groups are to work to their full potential. Whilst the role of the facilitator is challenging, inviting unpredictable learning areas, midwives should consider the benefits of progressing toward the philosophy of learning which is synonymous with current midwifery practice.
- Many theorists over the last century have assumed that groups pass through several stages as they develop. Understanding the stages of development may enhance the facilitator's ability to support the process of development without feeling a sense of failure during moments of tension and conflict. The stages involved in group development are: forming, storming, norming, performing and adjourning.
- Antenatal groups encourage the development of social support networks, the benefits of which are well established. Resource commitment from NHS trusts and local health agencies would secure the progress and quality of antenatal education into the 21st century.
- Preparation through antenatal education may enable partners to progress through the birth and postnatal experience feeling empowered to be able to offer support.
- A valuable part of antenatal education is the evaluation. The aim and nature of the evaluation will determine when and how it is carried out. It is useful for midwives to formalise methods of evaluation to enable audit and provision of data, which demonstrate the viability of the programme.

References

Bales R F, Cohen S P, Williamson S A 1979 A system for the multiple level observation of groups. Free Press, New York

Bloom B 1956 Taxonomy of education objectives: the classification of educational goals, handbook 1 cognitive domain. McKay, New York

Child D 1993 Psychology and the teacher. Cassell, London

Ewles L, Simnett I 1999 Promoting health: a practical guide, 4th edn. Baillière Tindall, London

Festinger L 1950 Informal social communication. Psychological Review 57:271–282

Fisher R, Wry W 1981 Getting to yes: negotiating agreement without giving in. Houghton-Mifflin, Boston MA

Forsyth D R 1990 Group dynamics, 2nd edn. Brooks Cole, Pacific Grove CA, p 13

Hill W F, Gruner L 1973 A study of development in open and closed groups. Small Group Behaviour 4:355–381

Hillan E M 1992 Issues in the delivery of midwifery care. Journal of Advanced Nursing 17:274–278

Julkunen K, Liukkonen A 1998 Fathers' experiences of childbirth. Midwifery 14:10–17

Knowles M 1990 The adult learner a neglected species, 4th edn. Gulf, Houston TX

Knowles M, Holton E, Swanson R 1998 The adult learner. Gulf, Houston TX

Leap N 1991 Helping you to make your own decisions: antenatal and postnatal groups in Deptford, SE London (VHS video)

Leery M R 1983 Understanding social anxiety. Sage, Newbury Park CA

Lewin K 1951 Field theory in social science. Harper, New York

Miller B 1994 Client education theory and practice. Mosby, New York

Nolan M 1998 Antenatal education, a dynamic approach. Baillière Tindall, London

O'Meara C 1993 An evaluation of consumer perspectives of childbirth and parenting education. Midwifery 9:210–219

Okpala D 1991 Preventing postnatal depression. Nursing Standard 5 (36):32–34

Quinn F 1995 The principles and practice of nurse education. Chapman & Hall, London

Raphael-Leff J 1993 Psychological processes of childbearing. Chapman & Hall, London

Rogers C, Freiberg H J 1994 Freedom to learn. Macmillan, New York

Schott J, Priest J 1991 Leading antenatal classes, a practical guide. Butterworth-Heinemann, Oxford

Shambaugh P W 1978 The development of the small group. Human Relations 31:283–295

Slavin R 1988 Educational psychology, theory into practice, 2nd edn. Prentice Hall, Englewood Cliffs NJ

Szeverenyi P, Poka R, Rorok Z 1998 Contents of childbirth-related fear among couples wishing the partner's presence at delivery. Journal of Psychosomatic Obstetrics and Gynaecology 19(1):38–43

Tuckman B W 1965 Developmental sequences in small groups. Psychological Bulletin 63:384–399

Tuckman B W, Jenson M A C 1977 Stages of small group development. Group and Organisational Studies 2:4–10

Wolf S 1985 Manifest and latent influence of majorities and minorities. Journal of Personality and Social Psychology 48:899–908

Recommended reading

Bond L A, Burns C 1998 Investing in parents' development as an investment in primary prevention. Journal of Mental Health 7(5):493–503

This paper offers an extensive and alternative view to parenting.

Nolan M 1998 Antenatal education: a dynamic approach. Baillière Tindall, London

A practical approach to antenatal education offers useful tips for childbirth educators.

11 Evaluating health promotion activities

Key themes

- The meaning of evaluation
- Why evaluate?
- Process, impact and outcome evaluation
- Process evaluation in action, a midwifery initiative
- Measures/methods
- Ethical considerations

Overview

This chapter aims to encourage the reader to explore the meaning of evaluation and consider its importance in relation to health promotion. Evaluation is explored in terms of process, outcome and impact, with reference made to the significance of subjective health measures. Midwifery examples are used to illustrate and explain different evaluation designs. A more detailed approach to evaluation is beyond the scope of this chapter. The reader is encouraged to utilise complementary texts from the recommended reading list.

Reflection points

- Consider health promotion activities that you have evaluated to date. This may be a small scale evaluation carried out at the end of, for example, a breast-feeding workshop or a research project.

The meaning of evaluation

Evaluation is the formation of criteria by which to determine the value of an idea or a method. The purpose of this is to demonstrate the success or failure of the method based on its aims and objectives (Downie, Tannahill & Tannahill 1996). The literal meaning of evaluation is to assess whether an idea or method is of value or importance. Generally each stakeholder will utilise the evaluation output toward a predetermined goal. The fundholders of a project will undoubtedly place value on the success of the activity in relation to cost effectiveness. Individuals involved in the programme delivery may consider raising public awareness and encouraging people to make choices as determinants of value. The scope of evaluation is far broader than the measurement of aims and objectives. Generally health education programmes encourage a number of other consequences, which can be measured against a standard or an indicator of good performance. Effective evaluation is not purely determined by measurable outcome, but process evaluation is of equal importance and is discussed later. Evaluation should have a clear aim and be relevant to the aims and objectives of the study, ensuring that the resources invested in the process of evaluation are worthwhile.

- What were the aims and objectives of the evaluation?
- What were the results of the evaluation and how were they used?

Why would you evaluate your health promotion programme?

Evaluation of health promotion programmes provides data which will influence future programmes, with regards to their method of delivery, content and process, as well as helping people to decide whether the programme should be replicated, modified, continued or discarded. Ultimately evaluation is concerned with assessing effectiveness and efficiency. This is sometimes difficult to measure, particularly if the aim of the activity is to influence feeling and emotion, which present a wide range of subjective variation.

Evaluation serves to:

- judge the success of a programme in relation to its defined objectives
- inform you of how well you carried out the activity
- highlight areas where improvement may be needed
- help other midwives by producing a description of the programme for replication (see next section, Process evaluation)
- justify the use of resources needed to carry out the activity
- make decisions about how resources will be allocated
- identify any unplanned or unexpected outcomes
- ensure ethical practice
- improve knowledge and understanding of cause and effect in interventions (Holman, Donovan & Corti 1993).

The benefits and value of evaluating a health promotion programme are that this not only demonstrates the effectiveness of a programme but also provides a learning opportunity for the health promoter. Reflective practice can be informed by evaluation, and assist in the personal and professional development of the health promoter. This will encourage the maintenance of high standards of practice and performance. All too often evaluation is viewed as a painful experience to be avoided. This may be more apparent toward the completion of individual antenatal classes. Failure to carry out an evaluation may provide the individual with short term psychological comfort, but lead to long term incompetence. The effectiveness of health

Discussion questions

- How would you ensure that your evaluation findings were disseminated to the stakeholders and other related parties?
- What factors need to be considered when preparing evaluation results for presentation to peer groups, stakeholders and other interested parties?

promotion work can be taken seriously, only if rigorous evaluation is conducted. Midwives are frequently involved in valuable health promotion work which has an impact on the mother and baby, but cannot be demonstrated by evaluation data. Evaluation involving anecdotal feedback is not useful in determining validity. Outputs must be evaluated to demonstrate the effectiveness and efficiency of the activity. Repeating a programme without assessing its effectiveness may disguise futile activities, wasting time and resources. Evaluation has the potential to inform plans of health promotion programmes by identifying successes and failures and adding to the growing knowledge base of practice (Naidoo & Wills 1994).

So far it is clear that evaluation data serve a purpose for the health promoter and ultimately for the client. Other stakeholders, however, may include the employing NHS trust or health authority, which may be funding the programme or seeking to improve, reduce or remove funding from a particular programme. The evaluation process and method used should therefore be rigorous and robust to be able to meet the demands of all stakeholders and should form part of the planning stages of the programme.

Process, impact and outcome evaluation

The evaluation of a health promotion programme or activity should be explored, clarified and identified during the early stages of programme development. This will identify at the outset the strengths and weakness of intended measures and provide clarity and focus for the direction of the programme. Discovering toward the end of the programme that the results of variables measured are meaningless and cannot support the aim of the activity is a waste of time and resources, not to mention turmoil for those who are involved in the planning stages and other stakeholders of the programme. Evaluation involves process, impact and outcome measures, which collectively form output measures of health promotion activity.

Process evaluation

This is an in-depth examination of the operation of the programme, the aim of which is to provide descriptive information of how a programme is implemented and functions. It may be used to improve an ongoing or new programme. It also provides those who wish to replicate the programme, with a clear, detailed description. The knowledge that health promotion activities are effective at achieving the desired outcomes is not enough to reassure others of its total effectiveness, who may be interested in replication. The process involves the collection of both qualitative and quantitative data. Although this may be viewed as time consuming and detracting from the evaluation of programme outcomes, process evaluation provides details underlying fundamental issues about how the objectives were achieved. An example of this is a health promotion programme or initiative which is deemed successful, to the detriment of the health of staff who were involved in the programme delivery. The objectives of process evaluation may therefore identify this extremely important variable which has repercussions for repeatability of the programme. It may be highly inappropriate to repeat a programme which may produce the required health results for the public, but create large levels of sickness within the establishment, and present challenges to the moral and ethical principles of the programme process.

Process evaluation addresses the following questions (Polit & Hunglar 1991).

- Does the programme function as planned – that is the way the designers intended?
- What appear to be the strongest and weakest aspects of the programme?
- What exactly is the treatment and does it differ (if at all) from the traditional practices?
- What was the process by which the programme was shaped and became fully operational?
- What, if any, were the barriers to successfully implementing the programme?
- How have the staff dealt with these barriers?
- What factors facilitated the implementation process?
- What were the characteristics of the participants, the staff and the setting of the programme?
- Did the programme serve the clients for whom the programme was designed?
- How do staff and clients like the programme?
- Have there been any problems in recruiting people to participate in the programme?
- Have there been any problems with staff turnover?
- Have staff been adequately trained to implement the programme?
- If staff turnover has occurred has training for replacement staff been adequate?
- Can the programme be readily replicated in a new setting or was its implementation affected by something unique in the setting in which it first operated?

Methods used for process evaluation may include interviews, diaries, observation and content analysis of documents (Naidoo & Wills 1994).

Process evaluation in action – a midwifery initiative

Consider the idea of raising public awareness of preconception care, with the aim of encouraging attendance at a preconception care class (Table 11.1).

Table 11.1

Examples of issues addressed at preconception care classess

Health issue	Aim of activity/ programme	Objectives of activity or programme	Health promotion activity	Evaluation methods
Adequate intake of essential dietary nutrients for pregnant women	• To encourage women planning a pregnancy to eat a healthy diet	• Women will understand the basic principles of a healthy diet • Understand that healthy eating can be achieved at low budget cost • Propose an individual eating plan which reflects a healthy diet at low cost • Maintain a healthy-eating plan throughout the remainder of pregnancy	• Run a healthy-eating programme; venue preconception care class and/or 'early bird' class • Health education approach including self-empowerment and client-centred work: 1. discussion of personal daily diets 2. developing a healthy-eating plan 3. starting and maintaining a healthy-eating plan diary 4. follow-up support throughout the pregnancy	• Administration of pre- and post-test questionnaires to assess knowledge gained as a result of the healthy-eating programme • Daily diary entries reflecting eating plans • Administration of a questionnaire postdelivery to determine success
Folic acid supplement-ation during the preconception period	• To encourage women planning a pregnancy to take folic acid supplements	• Women understand the reason why prenatal folic acid supplementation is necessary • Women planning a pregnancy take folic acid supplementation	• Health education approach including self-empowerment and client-centred work: 1. discuss availability and accessibility 2. discuss dietary sources 3. encourage the development of strategies to ensure compliance 4. identify start date for taking folic acid supplementation	• Administration of pre- and post-test questionnaires to assess knowledge gained as a result of the programme • Assessment of uptake and maintenance by the distribution of a questionnaire and focused interview, possibly after the first trimester of pregnancy

Health issue	Aim of activity/ programme	Objectives of activity or programme	Health promotion activity	Evaluation methods	Table 11.1 *(cont'd)*
Smoking during pregnancy	• To enable pregnant women and their partners who wish to give up smoking to do so successfully	• Enhanced decision-making skills • Reduction in the number of pregnant women and their partners who smoke • Successful smoking cessation • Utilise damage limitation principles for those who continue smoking	• Health education approach including self-empowerment and client-centred work: 1. smoking cessation programme 2. utilisation of intervention methods 3. continuity of support person	• Administration of pre- and post-test questionnaires to assess knowledge gained as a result of the programme • Assessment of the change process by the completion of daily diaries • Administration of questionnaires postdelivery to assess compliance and 6 months after that to assess maintenance • Focused interview, 6 months after the delivery date, to understand the process of compliance or non-compliance	
Alcohol and its detrimental effects on the fetus	• To raise awareness of the effects of alcohol consumption prenatally and antenatally for both the woman and her partner	• Enabling couples to understand the teratogenic effects of alcohol on their ability to conceive and on the fetus if conception occurs • A reduction in the number of couples who drink alcohol 6 months prior to conception	• Alcohol awareness programme: provision of evidence-based information, interactive teaching and learning methods • Identify 'risky' drinking behaviour Counsel and advise toward abstinence	• Administration of pre- and post-test questionnaires to assess knowledge gained as a result of the programme • Administration of a questionnaire after the delivery of the baby to test compliance • Focused interview after the delivery date to understand the process of compliance or non-compliance	

The target group may be women of childbearing age and their partners. Midwives may choose to market this initiative in a public arena to achieve maximum impact. A busy shopping centre may be the forum of choice, after market research identifies a high percentage of users and permission for use is granted by the owners. The primary intent of this initiative, in this situation, may be to raise public awareness generally about preconception care, and the secondary intent is to encourage attendance to the preconception care programme for those people who are planning to have a baby in the foreseeable future. The evaluation then would focus on the number of people who signed up for the programme as a result of the primary intent of this activity. Formal sign-up procedures would identify the characteristics and numbers of those who wished to attend the programme, but individual intent does not always determine behavioural commitment. Commitment to attend should therefore be demonstrated by actual attendance on the day. Difficulty arises when trying to assess the number of people who were made aware of the initiative but chose not to engage on the preconception care programme. At this time one can only speculate that they became more aware and chose to do nothing else with the information, they became more aware and decided to tell friends and family, or they became more aware and decided to make a lifestyle change, for example take folic acid supplementation, eat a healthier diet and seek advice about smoking cessation. Whether the improved behaviour is as a result of the campaign is pure conjecture and would warrant a rigorous research design to establish an association. Obtaining data about non-participants (i.e. those who did not acknowledge the initiative) is very difficult. Precise information about numbers and individuals who became aware of the programme can be gained from population-based surveys, but this would be an expensive strategy for collecting data.

Evaluation is planned to answer the question: Is the programme reaching its target audience? Questions for consideration may include:

• Is the shopping centre the best place to target men and women of childbearing age?
• At what time of the day did the initiative take place?
• On what day did the initiative take place?
• Was the initiative accessible, visibly appealing, inviting and non-threatening?
• Were the materials used to convey the message appropriate?
• Was the information tailored to meet the cultural needs of that particular community?
• Was the information accurate; was the language appropriate?

The secondary intent of the initiative is to encourage attendance to the preconception care programme for those people who are planning to have a baby in the foreseeable future. Process evaluation will measure if the programme is having the effect it is designed to have. Although this is primarily concerned with outcomes, the effects can be conceptualised as a chain of events leading from the start of the programme to the ultimate outcome (Downie, Tannahill & Tannahill 1996). For example, the preconception care programme may have increased knowledge and awareness, explored strategies that would enable the adoption of health principles, empowered individuals to make healthy lifestyle choices, encouraged a change in dietary intake and encouraged the cessation of smoking and other social poisons. The various effects that the programme has on the participants can be thus used as measurable outcomes for evaluation. The outcome of the programme could therefore be assessed using one or more of these variables. The appropriate variable to demonstrate the outcome of the programme can be largely determined to a certain extent on the available scientific evidence which has established causal links between one variable and another. For example, as there is over-whelming evidence to suggest that taking folic acid supplements reduces the incidence of neural tube defects in the developing fetus (MRC 1991), it may be useful to measure the uptake of folic acid as a supplement and the outcome as a result of supplementation. It may, however, be more beneficial to the organisation if several outcomes were measured to demonstrate the plausibility of the programme.

Impact evaluation

This type of evaluation is concerned with the immediate effects of the programme. It is an extremely popular type of evaluation used at the end of an antenatal education class. Midwives may choose to assess the participants' knowledge base and determine whether they feel that the programme may influence their future behaviour. It is important to acknowledge that this approach assesses information based on the participants' perception of their future behaviour. If this is the intention of the programme then the objectives would be measured accordingly. Consideration should be given to evaluation methods which assess knowledge and information processing from this premise. Impact evaluation which assesses behavioural change may demonstrate short term effects, and does not determine long term success. Impact evaluation may assess the impact of the programme in terms of raised awareness of a particular issue or the provision of new knowledge. Women who attend a breast-feeding workshop, for example, may feel a strong desire to breast feed, owing to the impact of the programme. If this was the objective of the activity, then the objective would have been achieved. This would not determine long term influence. Other areas easily measured at this time may be the appropriateness of visual aids and other learning methods used by the facilitator.

Outcome evaluation

As the name suggests, outcome evaluation is concerned with outcome measures of effectiveness of the programme against the objectives set. It is concerned with the long term consequences. Evaluation of an antenatal education programme, for example, may assess the outcome of the programme, 6 weeks after the birth of the baby at the postnatal reunion class. This forum creates an opportunity for discussion about birth experiences and in addition is often used to evaluate the usefulness of health issues taught antenatally. Parents at the postnatal reunion may inform the midwife that they had put the principles taught antenatally into practice; for example, clients may have utilised the relaxation principles during labour and the postnatal period and continue to use relaxation as a part of their everyday lives, or they may feel that the session on breast feeding reinforced their breast feeding skills and had a positive influence on their uptake and continuation. The methods by which this information may be collected is explored later. The effectiveness of the programme should, however, be measured by utilising reliable techniques and an appropriate evaluation design.

A further example of outcome evaluation can be demonstrated by referring to Table 11.1. Within a preconception care programme, pregnant women and their partners who smoke are expected to stop smoking as a result of smoking cessation and intervention counselling (also see Ch. 6). Assessing the number of participants who smoke and the number of cigarettes smoked per day at the start of a smoking cessation programme and comparing this data with data collected, for example, 6 months after the completion of the programme is an example of a small scale outcome evaluation. The methods of data collection (see Table 11.1) are both quantitative and qualitative. The results would demonstrate the number of participants who had continued to smoke and those who had stopped and the reasons why. However, if control for chance factors and influencing variables which impressed upon the smoking behaviour were not included in the design of the study, the effectiveness of the intervention would be seriously questioned. Consideration should, therefore, be given to variables which may have influenced the cessation of smoking other than the content of the programme. A control group, by way of comparison, of those who had not attended the programme (see Ch. 6) would therefore present a more accurate picture of the reliability of the intervention. Preconception classes at present are not routinely available within the NHS. The availability of programmes is sparse and, as such, clients attending are therefore more likely to be motivated toward and receptive to adopting healthy lifestyles. Compliance to adjust to healthy behaviours will therefore be high. This is a useful factor to consider during planning stages of the programme.

Large scale outcome evaluation identifies the effectiveness of an intervention or programme and, as such, requires rigorous methods to demonstrate that the effects are attributed exclusively to the intervention and not to other factors.

Objectives of the programme activity

Understanding the meaning of objectives will help to clarify the process required for measurement. Objectives are criteria by which the desired outcomes of the programme are assessed. They also help the direction and planning of the programme. A useful approach for objective setting for antenatal education can involve informing clients of the objectives of the programme and encouraging them to set their own learning objectives. This helps to enforce a sense of client autonomy, commitment and owner-ship of the programme. An approach considered to be more scientific involves objectives which are specific to the aim of the programme and may not measure incidental programme output.

The objectives in Table 11.1 are a combination of psychomotor objectives (what the clients do – skills based), cognitive objectives (what the clients know – knowledge based) and affective objectives (what the clients feel – attitudes based). It is essential that health promotion activities do not purely concentrate on behavioural outcome. Understanding the process behind a particular behavioural change in relation to the influences of the client's thoughts, feelings and socioeconomic and cultural identity will undoubtedly assist the health promoter in beginning to understand the complex process of compliance and non-compliance. Hence there is a need to set objectives which represent influencing health and behavioural factors. During the planning stages of the programme consideration should be given to how each objective set will be measured. Continuing with the examples in Table 11.1, the methods used to assess the achievement of objectives are questionnaire, daily dairies and focused interview. When choosing a method of data collection which will determine the achievement of the objective, consideration should be given to the appropriateness of the method, in relation to the depth and quality of information that is achievable by the method of data collection chosen. The example from Table 11.1, encouraging a healthy diet during the preconception period, will help to illustrate this point. The aim is to encourage women planning a pregnancy to eat a healthy diet. As mentioned above, the objectives are psychomotor, cognitive and affective in nature. The methods chosen to evaluate the objectives are questionnaire, which will measure compliance, and focus interview, which will help to identify reasons for compliance, non-compliance and to explore thoughts and feelings about the whole process. The content of the focus interview, however, is largely determined by the topic guide used (see interview technique). In this example self-empowerment is not a stated objective but the process of the activity strengthens the skills and capabilities of the individual to take action and control by developing an eating plan and adjusting their diet accordingly. In this particular example therefore, empowerment, although not directly measured, is a valued outcome.

Measures/methods

There are a vast range of evaluation approaches which are used in health promotion. These include randomised control trials, survey techniques and observational studies.

Given the wide range of health promotion activities integral to the midwife's role, an equally wide range of evaluation methods is required. It is important to bear in mind, however, that the output measures (process, impact and outcome) should assess the various components of health and not purely a single value which highlights a limited definition of health. Chapter 1 explored the concept of health and concluded that physical, mental, emotional, societal, spiritual and social aspects of health are all interrelated and interdependent, fostering the view that health is an holistic concept. For the purpose of evaluation of health promotion initiatives, health indicators should reflect the holistic view of health and ill health in order for output to present the whole picture of effectiveness. Health profiles, as defined by Hunt, McEwen & McKenna (1986), comprise an example of a health indicator which clearly acknowledges different aspects of health, without aggregation to a single value: disparate measures, for example pain and social support, are given their own value as opposed to being aggregated. In contrast, the McMaster health index questionnaire produces a health index by aggregating scores derived from 59 questions, measured by criteria ranging from good function response to poor function response, based on physical function items, social function items and emotional function items (Chambers et al 1976). The potential to lose valuable information is more likely using this questionnaire. The Quality-adjusted life cycle (QUALY) is an example of an outcome health indicator. It measures how many years of life are added as a result of medical interventions and how the intervention has improved the quality of life (Paton 1996). This may include, for example, assessing the outcome of smoking cessation programmes or breast-feeding workshops. Questions may include: Are the outcomes worthwhile? and are they cost effective? QUALY is concerned with outcomes and how they relate to cost. As such, it is considered to be a sensitive, effective method of determining resource allocation within the health service and is commonly used by health economists. The QUALY acknowledges that adding years to life is not synonymous with adding quality, however. There is also cause for concern about using the QUALY as a health indicator when decisions and judgements are removed from those who are a part of the service and are expert practitioners within the service (Smith 1987). Within health promotion the use of health indicators which enable subjective measures are more appropriate than the QUALY, and conducive to the woman-centred approach to midwifery care.

It is essential that evaluation designs are tailored to suit the activity of the programme (see Box 11.1). Combining different research methodologies presents the advantage of eliciting not only quantifiable data, but also findings which enable the expression of thoughts, feelings and exploration of meaning, which clearly differ from biochemical, microbiological and mortality indices (see Table 11.1).

Interviews

Focused interview

This method involves the interviewer and the respondent. A prepared topic guide may be used by the interviewer to provide focus and specifies the wording of all questions to be asked during the interview with each client. The client is encouraged to talk freely about all subjects or questions on the topic guide. The responses may be recorded on a tape recorder. This method is useful for collecting qualitative data – that is, data which represent individuals' thoughts, feelings and opinions, within the context of their own experience. It is a useful way for the evaluator to explore areas in great detail. It is, however, time consuming as responses need to be analysed and themed to elicit a conclusion. Unfortunately also, some clients may feel intimidated by the experience of being interviewed and may not speak freely, honestly and spontaneously.

Focus group interview

This type of interview involves a small group of people brought together

---

Box 11.1 **Case scenario: Kemi**

Kemi has successfully taught antenatal and postnatal exercises for the past 3 years. She determined success based on criteria of compliance to perform the exercise, and to do so correctly, and longevity of the activity. To establish the results Kemi telephoned her clients and asked questions based on her success criteria. She recorded all information in her teaching portfolio.

Reflection points

- What are the strengths and weaknesses of the evaluation in terms of process, impact and outcome?

- What improvements could be made?

for a group discussion. The discussion is led by the interviewer who may use a series of questions or a topic guide to focus discussion. This method benefits the interviewer, in that the views and opinions of a group of people can be obtained in a short space of time. Although this method is less time consuming than individual interviews, group members who feel unable to speak freely in groups may not have their opinions heard. Even with good facilitation some members of the group may feel intimidated by others and therefore not express their view; alternatively they may comply with what appears to be the status quo.

Both individual and group interviews may be reconvened some time after the health promotion activity to assess long term impact. They also enable the interviewer to assess the clients' level of understanding of the questions or statements posed, by observing verbal/non-verbal behaviour. The same question therefore can be repeated in a different way in order to correct misunderstandings. Interviewees with literacy and language problems are more able to respond to questions using the interview method of data collection, more so than methods which require reading and written responses. In summary, despite the many benefits of the interview method, certain disadvantages are apparent. Interview methods are time consuming and expensive. Available resources will determine whether this method of evaluation is justifiable

Questionnaires

Questionnaires are effective at collecting large amounts of information at low cost. They also offer complete anonymity, which increases the response rate. Questionnaires can be self administered, group administered or postal. Each has its own advantages and disadvantages and should be chosen in relation to the purpose and appropriateness. Individual bias can, to a large extent, be avoided but not totally eradicated. Once the respondents receive the questionnaire their views and/or stereotypes of the organisation or the individual who carried out the programme may influence their responses (Oppenheim 1992). Questionnaires are made up of open-ended and closed questions. Closed questions usually offer respondents a choice of replies, which they identify usually by ticking the response which best suits their answer. Open-ended questions invite a free, spontaneous response. Closed questions offer no room for exploration or depth of a response, whilst open-ended questions allow clients to respond in their own words. This too can pose problems with individuals who do not, or indeed cannot, formalise a response, are illiterate or visually impaired, or to whom the presented language is a barrier. There is no opportunity to correct misunderstandings and control the way the question is answered. Generally the questionnaire method invites more of a superficial response than the interview technique, but is more cost effective in relation to time factors and analysis of the findings.

Surveys

The two common types of survey are descriptive and analytical. Descriptive surveys are involved with counting either a representative sample of the population, in which case inferences can be made about the remainder of the population, or the whole population. Either way, a descriptive survey provides information about the proportion of the population who perform a certain task, or who have a certain opinion. It does not explain behaviour nor show causal relationships. Descriptive surveys have been used successfully by the Office of National Statistics to inform social trends and by the government prior to taking political action. Surveys with an analytic design are able to determine why things happen through analysis of causality.

The survey method can be a useful evaluation tool for midwives to utilise for small health promotion initiatives or antenatal education, but it does require well-formulated questions and an understanding that conclusions can be drawn only about the group to which the intervention was intended. To generalise findings, an appropriate research design would need to be formulated.

Reliability and validity

The reliability and validity of questions in the above methods present a challenge to their developmental process when used in large project evaluation. Each question is supposed to measure a particular variable and, as such, if the measure were repeated the same results would be established. Reliability is therefore concerned with consistency and repeatability of a measure – that is, the probability of achieving the same result if duplicated. Validity determines whether a question, or item, measures what it is supposed to measure.

Daily diaries

Clients may be asked to spend 5 minutes a day writing down their thoughts about the intervention; alternatively, they may be given a structure or outline to follow when completing their daily accounts

This method of evaluation enables the evaluator to follow the client's progress of behaviour, thoughts and feelings in relation to the assessed intervention. It relies on an assumption that respondents have literacy skills, an ability to express themselves against the criteria set, memory recall and commitment to complete daily accounts as contemporaneously as possible to ensure accuracy.

This technique is, however, difficult to design and analyse, the analysis and interpretation being extremely time consuming.

Performance indicators

Many organisations, particularly the NHS, use performance indicators to measure and monitor activity. The technique is particularly useful when seeking to define success of an intervention, policy or strategy. Performance indicators may also be viewed as standards by which current provision of care is assessed and are commonly referred to as targets by which to measure success. A performance indicator therefore seeks to illustrate the success of an objective in terms of when the objective should be achieved and the quantity and the quality of the achievement. For example, the document, Our healthier nation, saving lives (Secretary of State for Health 1999) uses this approach in its national strategy for health. One of five overall targets includes: 'To reduce the death rate by cancer amongst people aged under 65 years by at least a further fifth (20%) by 2010' (p. 57). To reach this target it is proposed that the government, health authorities, health agencies and the community play a part in tackling factors which predispose to death from cancer. A multiagency approach with resource allocation and appropriate timing renders the target achievable.

Stott, Kinnersley & Rollnick (1994) suggest that unrealistic targets and the pressure to produce results can cause health professionals to feel bullied or bribed by the government to achieve targets that many clients are not ready to accept for personal and social reasons. The cost to the relationship between the client and the professional, and the feelings of integrity and self-respect, can be somewhat overlooked in the drive to achieve the target set. Performance indicators should therefore be realistic in relation to timing, quantity and quality. Resources are a major influence on the achievement of the performance indicator and should be taken into consideration. Unrealistic performance indicators apply pressure on health promoters to meet the indicator by the quickest means.

Ethical considerations

The basic ethical principle regarding methods of data collection is that respondents should suffer no harm from their involvement throughout the evaluation process. Respecting the autonomy of clients, whether or not they comply with the evaluation process, is paramount. Their right to privacy and any refusal to respond to questions should also be respected. The intentions of output evaluation should be integral to the aim of the programme and should be used accordingly. The results of evaluations which are not utilised, question the aim of the programme.

Summary

- Evaluation is a dynamic and ongoing process. It provides the means for demonstrating effective and efficient health promotion activities and encourages the development of reflective evidence-based practice. Knowledge gained through evaluation provides a knowledge base for other practitioners to monopolise on the strengths and weaknesses of that approach.
- A clear focus on the evaluation process during the planning stages of the health promotion programme with an identification of measurable outcomes will undoubtedly reduce complications toward the end of the programme.
- Pre-experimental evaluation designs are utilised frequently by midwives to evaluate small scale evaluation activities. Experimental designs, however, are used to determine cause and effect and require extensive knowledge and understanding of the research process. Whichever the design utilised, demonstrating a rigorous and robust evaluation strategy formalises health promotion activities.
- The different types of evaluation provide information about different aspects of a given programme. Process evaluation enables replication of a study or part of a study, impact evaluation informs of immediate effects and outcome evaluation demonstrates the efficiency of interventions, programmes or activities. Process, impact and outcome evaluation together constitute output.
- The varied methods used for evaluation provide qualitative and quantitative data which demonstrate the achievement of the objectives of the programme and can be utilised when addressing the cost effectiveness of the activity.
- An important point to remember is that evaluation is worthwhile only if it can make a difference. Evaluation results are not useful if they are not interpreted, utilised and presented, and the exercise becomes futile.
- Practitioners may use the results of the evaluation to support their personal and professional development, develop new standards of practice or support existing standards and encourage reflective evidence-based practice. The results may also encourage the influx of further funds into the programme.

References

Chambers L W, Sackett D L, Godsmith C H, Macpherson A S 1976 Development and application of an index of social function. Health Services Research 11:18–20

Crookes P, Davies S 1998 Research into practice. Baillière Tindall, Edinburgh

Downie R S, Tannahill C, Tannahill A 1996 Health promotion: models and values. Oxford University Press, New York

Holman C D J, Donovan R T, Corti B 1993 Evaluating projects funded by the West Australian Health Promotion Foundation: a systematic approach. Health Promotion International 8:199–208

Hunt S M, McEwen J, McKenna S P 1986 Measuring health status. Croom Helm, London

Medical Research Council (MRC) Vitamin Study Research Group 1991 Prevention of neural tube defects, results of the Medical Research Council vitamin study. Lancet 338:131–137

Naidoo J, Wills J 1994 Health promotion foundations for practice. Baillière Tindall, London

Oppenheim A N 1992 Questionnaire design, interviewing and attitude measurement. Printer, London

Paton C 1996 Health policy and management. The healthcare agenda in a British political context. Chapman & Hall, London

Polit D, Hunglar B 1991 Nursing research principles and methods. J B Lippincott, Philadelphia

Secretary of State for Health 1999 Our healthier nation, saving lives. The Stationery Office, London

Smith A 1987 Qualms about QUALYs. Lancet 1:1134–1136

Stott N C, Kinnersley P, Rollnick S 1994 The limits to health promotion. British Medical Journal 309:971–972

Recommended reading

Gilbert N 1998 Researching social life. Sage, London

Nutbeam D 1998 Evaluating health promotion – progress, problems and solutions. Health Promotion International 13(1):27–43
This paper presents the difficulties of evaluating health promotion activites.

Polger S, Thomas S 1995 Introduction to research in the health sciences, 3rd edn. Longman, Harlow, Essex
A useful text which provides a foundation for evaluation research.

Rees C 1997 An introduction to research for midwives. Books for Midwives Press, Cheshire

Smith P 1997 Research mindedness for practice. An interactive approach for nursing and health care. Churchill Livingstone, New York

Index